Stop Negative Thinking

The Step-by-Step Plan

to Overcome Negativity And Stop Overthinking.

Declutter Your Mind and Start Thinking Positively Now.

Anita Allen

What is Negative Thinking?

It was already mentioned in the introduction but it bears repeating: negative thoughts are normal. We cannot escape the occasional low mood, worry, or gloomy thought. In fact, trying to ban all negativity from our lives just creates more negative stress because it puts unrealistic pressure on ourselves. It's perfectly natural to experience worry if you suddenly lose your job or to feel annoyed if your neighbors keep throwing loud parties late into the night. It's when you begin to fixate solely on these thoughts and feelings that they become a problem. In the context of this book, the phrase "negative thinking" doesn't refer to occasional passing thoughts or worry over one-off stressful situations, but rather to the habit of repetitive, persistent, pervasive negative thinking. This could come in the form of constantly replaying past events or conversations, overanalyzing, beating yourself up, fixating on a situation, or worrying obsessively about the future. People struggling with this habit might think negatively about themselves, others, or the world around them in general. Whatever form their negative thoughts take, however, eventually the habit will begin to seriously impact their lives.

Negative thinking can be sneaky as well. It can creep up on you without you really noticing it until suddenly, negative thoughts hold sway over your day or even your life. After all, no one sets out to develop a bad habit; it happens gradually over time and in subtle ways. We often get so caught up in our day to-day lives that we rarely take the time to stop and really look at our thoughts. As a result, it is easy to engage in repetitive negative thinking without even realizing it. You might just notice that you're in a bad mood or that you feel "off" but upon closer examination, you realize that you've been mentally rehashing a recent fight with your mother all day.

Guilty Thinking

When a person is caught up in guilty thinking, they often find themselves trapped in the past. They feel guilty for mistakes they have made, replaying them over and over again. Perhaps you said something in anger that hurt your spouse's feelings; while it's normal to feel remorse in this situation, a habitual negative thinker will continue to beat themselves up for their words and feel crippling guilt even after they've apologized to their spouse. Another common example is making a mistake at work. Perhaps you input an incorrect number on a report, resulting in embarrassment in front of your boss or in extra work needed from yourself or your colleagues to fix the error. We all make mistakes, but negative thinkers will be unable to let it go. They'll replay it over and over, beating themselves up and telling themselves things like, "I can't believe I didn't double-check those numbers. I'm such an idiot.

I should never have volunteered to write that report. That meeting was so embarrassing, I looked like an incompetent screw-up. Heck, maybe I am!"

Guilty thinking often goes hand-in-hand with "shoulding" all-or-nothing thinking, and predicting the future.

Shoulding

This line of negative thinking happens when a person obsesses over what they "should" or "should not" do. In the previous example about the error at work, the person slipped into "should" thinking by telling themselves that they should have been more careful or that they should not have volunteered for the job. Perhaps you have been unhappy with your physical fitness and find yourself constantly thinking, "I shouldn't have eaten that. I should have gone to the gym today." While setting goals is admirable and important for our continued personal growth, constantly lecturing ourselves for things we have or have not done—or "shoulding on ourselves", in the words of motivational speaker Loretta Laroche (Laroche, 2008)—can be counterproductive to those goals. Instead of inspiring and motivating us, it just makes us feel worse about ourselves.

Should thinking often overlaps with guilty thinking, predicting the future, and mind reading.

All-or-Nothing Thinking

Always. Never. Every time. A person who finds themselves using words like these on a regular basis may be caught up in all-or-nothing thinking. If you are an all-or-nothing thinker, you see the world in black and white. Things are either good or bad. A certain aspect of your life always goes well or goes horribly. You are either perfect at something or a failure. So, how is this line of thinking negative? It leaves no room for normal human error or for happenstance. Say you are single and go out on a first date that doesn't go very well. If you are an all-or-nothing thinker, you might tell yourself, "I always screw up dating so why even bother trying? Relationships just never work out for me." Similarly, if you have a bad experience at a restaurant, you might think, "You can never find good customer service anymore. Society is just failing." This line of thinking ultimately lowers your level of regard for yourself and for the people around you.

All-or-nothing thinking often relates to worst case scenario thinking, predicting the future, and overall pessimism.

Worst Case Scenario Thinking/Worrying

Otherwise known as "catastrophizing" (Grohol, 2018), worst case scenario thinking or worrying happens when we believe in the worst possible outcome for a given situation. Recall our earlier example of an error at work. If you engage in worst case scenario thinking, you might worry and think, "I can't believe I made such a stupid mistake. I'm obviously going to get fired now." Perhaps you have a splitting headache and immediately think, "It must be a brain tumor." Similarly, perhaps a loved one is a bit late in contacting you and you start thinking, "There must have been a terrible accident." Clearly, such thinking can induce severe worry or even anxiety, particularly if it's a constant pattern.

Worst case scenario thinking often goes hand-in-hand with all-or-nothing thinking, predicting the future, and mind reading.

Predicting the Future

This line of negative thinking is very similar to worst case scenario thinking but it relates specifically to events and situations in the future. If you engage in this type of negative thinking, you view the potential for future happiness or success as very low. We could also call this "why bother" thinking. Imagine you line up an interview for your dream job; if you are caught in a pattern of predicting the future negatively, you might think, "I know I'm just going to be awkward and screw it up. Why should I even bother going?" Predicting-the-future thinking can influence your relationships as well. Perhaps you have moved to a new city and are invited to a party; your negative thought pattern might have you believe that people won't like you so you shouldn't attend.

Predicting the future thinking relates closely to worst case scenario thinking, all-or-nothing thinking, and overall pessimism. The future is always uncertain. Giving it certainty is only going to cause you mental anguish.

Mind Reading

When you engage in mind reading, you believe that you know what other people are thinking. You make assumptions about people's beliefs, thoughts, and feelings—and those assumptions are typically negative. You might walk by a group of co-workers and hear them laughing and think that they must be talking about you. If a friend doesn't respond to your text message immediately, you might jump to the conclusion that she must be angry with you. This line of thinking can be particularly harmful for your relationships because it makes you automatically assume the worst about people.

Mind reading often goes hand-in-hand with predicting the future and worst case scenario thinking.

Blaming

Blaming comes in two varieties: self-blame and blame of others. People who self-blame feel that they are responsible for everything that goes wrong in their lives. From their company not landing a prospective client to a special dinner not turning out well to missing an appointment because of traffic, they will believe that it was all their fault. Holding yourself accountable and taking responsibility for your actions and behaviors is healthy, but self-blame takes this to an unhealthy level, leading to low self-esteem and feelings of failure. When people perpetually place the blame on others, on the other hand, they abdicate their responsibility for any role they might have played. Someone who blames others might complain about their overly chatty coworker who prevents them from getting their work done rather than taking responsibility for their own lack of productivity. Similarly, they might choose to complain daily about how other drivers make their commute so long rather than just accepting the reality that everyone is sitting in the same traffic. Blaming can negatively impact your relationships, as well as diminish your sense of control over your own life and your ability to accept life as it is.

Blaming goes hand-in-hand with all-or-nothing thinking and pessimism.

Comparing

Comparing ourselves to others and finding ourselves lacking is a very common form of negative thinking. Virtually everyone has experienced instances when their inner critic has piped up. People might compare their looks, their relationship status, their wealth, their career path, or their material belongings. They also might compare themselves to their friends and family or to complete strangers. Constant comparison can lead to an overall feeling of dissatisfaction with your life and lowered self-esteem.

Comparing often goes along with worst case scenario thinking and predicting the future.

Pessimism

This is too good to last. Life is just supposed to be hard. People can't be trusted. Nothing is certain but death and taxes. If you find yourself making statements like these often, you might be engaging in overall pessimistic thinking. When you have this mindset, you expect things to go poorly. You expect other people and yourself to let you down. You find it hard to accept or trust when good things happen. Some people who are deeply caught in pessimistic thinking can even begin to take pleasure in situations going awry because it validates their worldview.

Pessimism relates closely to worst case scenario thinking, predicting the future, and blaming.

What Causes Negative Thinking?

Have you ever wondered, "Why am I so negative?" Or perhaps a loved one has told you, "You need to look on the bright side more often." Where does negative thinking stem from? Why do some people look at life as a glass half full while others see it as half empty? Is it nature or nurture?

It's become a commonly accepted idea that we are born with our own natural happiness set point. This is the level of happiness that we experience regardless of what is happening in our lives; whether everything is going well or we are experiencing challenges, our happiness set point remains generally the same. In fact, it's been shown that even when people experience a significant positive event like winning the lottery or a significant negative event like a serious medical diagnosis, their happiness set point returns to its baseline after about a year (Bloom, 2017). If people have happiness set points, it stands to reason that we also have our own individual levels of positivity and negativity. So, it may be the case that some people are just more predisposed to negative thinking than others. This is the nature side of the coin.

Our early childhood experiences also impact our personalities, mindsets, and worldviews. If you were raised in a household where negative thinking was prevalent, you likely learned some of the same behaviors. Perhaps you had an overly critical parent, causing you to compare and judge yourself harshly later in life. A parent who frequently expressed pessimistic thoughts may have taught you that the world is harsh or that the cards are stacked against you. More traumatic childhood experiences, such as neglect or abandonment, can lead to negative thinking patterns as well. Someone who suffered early trauma may engage in worst case scenario thinking, finding it hard to trust other people or take their word. Clearly, nurture plays as large a part as nature in determining whether you will be plagued by negative thinking.

A pattern of negative thinking can also be caused by stressful life events beyond childhood. The end of a relationship, the loss of a job, or a health scare can all spark negative thoughts which if not addressed can soon spiral out of control into habitual pessimistic thinking. Negative thinking functions like a feedback loop: the more we focus our attention on what's going wrong in our lives or in the world, the worse we feel. And the worse we feel, the harder it will be to have a positive attitude. It becomes a vicious cycle and those grooves of negativity in our mental track just get deeper and deeper.

For some people, negative thinking can even develop into an addiction. People for whom negativity becomes an addiction derive a sort of pleasure from the habit. As mentioned earlier, pessimistic thoughts can be used as a way to validate a person's worldview. Similarly, negative thoughts can be used to cement a person's identity ("I'm always a victim") or to try to make sense of or control the world around them ("People are just bad, that's all there is to it.") (Colier, 2019).

So much for how the habit of negative thinking can develop. Where do the specific negative thoughts themselves come from? If you begin to pay attention to the content of your negative thoughts, you'll notice that they fall into one of two camps: anxiety or fear about the future or guilt or anger about the past. We all experience these feelings from time to time, but habitual negative thinkers dwell on the past or the future and find it hard or even impossible to let their thoughts go and focus on the present.

For many people, negative thinking crops up in specific situations or with specific people. You may experience negative thinking in the form of social anxiety. Perhaps you worry that people won't like you or are talking about you behind your back in social settings; you might also find yourself constantly comparing yourself to others or judging them harshly. Some people are plagued by negative thinking in their work environments; they might complain constantly about their boss, their coworkers, or their customers, or demand perfection from themselves and others. Negativity can crop up at home as well. Perhaps you find yourself constantly criticizing your family members; you might also be consumed with worry about the health and well-being of your family or feel like you need to "do it all" yourself and thus make yourself a martyr. Your negativity could center on your body image and looks, your finances, or politics and the general state of the world.

What Are the Effects of Negative Thinking?

Breaking a habit like negative thinking is hard, but truly comprehending the impact of habitual negative thinking can give you the motivation to make a change. You might not even realize all the ways in which constant negative thoughts are intruding on your life.

One major effect is fairly obvious right off the bat: negative thinking creates negative feelings. People who constantly think gloomy thoughts will often feel irritable, sad, angry, hopeless, anxious, or apathetic. Habitual negative thinking can even develop into a more serious mental health condition such as depression or anxiety disorder. The bottom line is that thinking gloomy thoughts makes you feel bad.

Constant negativity can take a toll on your physical health as well. For example, constant worrying can disrupt your sleep and keep you up at night, leaving you feeling drained of energy and unable to concentrate. When you are tired and lethargic, you might be less likely to exercise or make healthy food choices. The stress produced by constant negative thinking can also drive people to unhealthy coping mechanisms such as smoking cigarettes or drinking alcohol in excess. And the list of physical effects doesn't end there. Perpetual anxiety or anger can increase your blood pressure and impact your digestion. Constant stress, such as that brought on by worry and negativity, raises the levels of cortisol produced in the body; this in turn can lower your immune system's ability to fight off infections. Studies have even found that pessimism, cynicism, and depression can increase a person's chances of heart disease and stroke (Hoffman, 2015).

In addition to eroding both your mental and your physical health, perpetual negative thinking affects your life in many other ways as well. While it might not seem obvious, one area of your life that can be impacted by negative thinking is your finances. The feelings of sadness, hopelessness, or depression brought on by negative thinking might make it hard for you to focus at work, thus reducing your productivity and eventually even threatening your job security. Similarly, negative self-judgments could keep you stuck in menial or low-paying work and make you less likely to apply for more lucrative employment opportunities. Some people turn to shopping as a way to distract themselves from negative thoughts and make themselves feel better; this can lead to overspending or even a shopping addiction.

Over time, negative thinking patterns can damage relationships as well. Most people won't want to spend time with someone who constantly complains, criticizes, or belittles others. In fact, research suggests that just listening to another person complaining can actually have negative health impacts; the brain of the person listening releases stress hormones that can reduce cognitive functions and lead to overall greater levels of stress (Montenegro, 2015). If you are a perpetual negative thinker, you may find friends or romantic partners begin to pull away from you. Similarly, you might have trouble making new friends. Work relationships can also be challenged by constant negativity; your colleagues may be hesitant to involve you in group work or to help you out with a project. Being labeled as difficult at work can even threaten your job itself.

A negative mindset can prevent you from solving problems effectively. This might sound counterintuitive: after all, shouldn't thinking about your problems help you find solutions? The truth is, overanalyzing and ruminating on negative events or situations can lead to analysis paralysis, preventing you from ever taking any action at all to address your problems. Habitual negative thinkers tend to be close-minded as well, impeding their ability to think outside the box and see creative solutions. They also might be less likely to reach out to others for help or advice.

Finally, negativity begets more negativity. Remember the feedback loop mentioned earlier? You might have noticed how on days when you wake up on the wrong side of the bed, everything else seems to go wrong, too. You spill coffee on your favorite shirt. You stub your toe. You miss your bus and end up being late for work. Some people believe that you attract negative events and situations by putting out negative energy. However, it could just be that when you are focusing on the negative, that is what you will see. What we place our attention on grows. If you constantly fixate on what is going wrong in your life, you will be more likely to notice every little bad thing and less likely to notice the good things.

How Can I Silence Those Negative Thoughts?

In later, we'll discuss specific strategies and practices to help you tame that negative voice in your head. For now, though, simply focus on becoming aware of your negative thoughts. Take some time to examine what forms they typically take. Understanding the causes of your negative thinking can be an important first step in breaking the habit. We cannot change what we're not aware of.

For example, when you determine what type of negative thinker you are— worst case scenario thinker, blamer, all-or-nothing thinker—you'll begin to notice those thoughts more often as they crop up, providing the opportunity to consciously let them go. Similarly, if you realize you tend to think more negatively in certain situations (at work, with your spouse, etc.), you can begin to think of ways to shift those situations so that you can feel more positive about them. The more you understand your negative thinking patterns, the better prepared you will be to choose the right strategies and practices to help you change them.

You may want to keep a journal or take notes on your smartphone for a few days to help you track your thinking patterns. When you notice yourself caught in a negativity loop, take a moment to jot down some of the details about it. Where were you when the negative thoughts popped up? Who were you with and what were you doing? What form did your negative thoughts take? Were you focused on the past or the future? Did the negativity center on yourself or on external factors (other people, world events, etc.)? How do the negative thoughts make you feel emotionally and physically? Do you notice any tension, tightness, or clenching in your body?

Becoming more aware of your negative thoughts can be uncomfortable. For example, you may begin to see clearly how your negativity has hurt those around you. It can be unpleasant to realize that your behavior has been harmful but such a realization is the only way to make amends and move forward with new behaviors. Awareness is a necessary first step. Your habit of negative thinking did not develop overnight, so breaking the habit will not happen immediately either. In order to truly break the pattern and clear mental space for new habits, you need to be willing to examine your thoughts and work through any uncomfortable emotions or knowledge they may bring up.

Think of your negative thought pattern as a physical illness. In order to know how best to treat you, your doctor would first need to perform tests to determine what type of illness you had and where it stemmed from.

+

Why Your Brain Ia Hard Wired For Negativity?

The first thing we have to gain control over is berating ourselves for our negative thought patterns. All those people that have told you that you are just a negative person, and you aren't trying to be positive, are wrong. Science tells us that our brain is trained to pay more attention to our negative thoughts. To an extent, there is a good reason for this.

On the one hand, when we are stressed or feeling scared, our brain releases the hormones cortisol and adrenaline. These two hormones play a crucial role in the fight or flight response. The fight or flight response is what protects us from danger. If your child crosses the road, the first response is to grab their hand and probably shout at them because we fear an accident—even if no car is coming. On the other hand, too much cortisol can have numerous consequences on our health. Some of these include:

- Weight gain

- Acne

- Thinning skin

- Easy bruising

- Muscle weakness

- Severe fatigue

- High blood pressure

- Headaches

Increased blood pressure, headaches, weight gain, and severe anxiety are also symptoms of too much adrenaline. You are also more at risk of heart attacks and strokes. So, the release of cortisol and adrenaline is generally a good thing, but as soon as negative thinking becomes a serious issue, we are putting our health at risk.

There is another problem with an overactive fight or flight response. An increase in cortisol increases white matter in the brain. White matter is good for communication between the gray matter of the brain, but it's the gray matter that carries out processes. Gray matter is necessary to cope with stress effectively. When white matter dominates, along with increased stress and fear, it becomes harder for us to decipher complex problems.

Those who don't suffer from negative thinking might be able to take a step back and view situations from alternative perspectives. In our heightened states, this is much more difficult.

We also have to consider that although our brain is an organ, it acts like a muscle in the sense that it needs training. Through no fault of our own, our brain has been trained in the wrong way. Our negative thoughts are processed in the right prefrontal cortex, just above your right eye. On the top, left-hand side of the brain, we have the left prefrontal cortex.

Thanks to technology that scans the brain, we can see that people who suffer from depression have an overdeveloped right prefrontal cortex and an underdeveloped left prefrontal cortex. Imagine lifting weights with only your right arm—your left will never be able to keep up.

But as the brain is not a muscle, how does this actually work? The brain contains approximately 100 billion neurons, and each neuron has an average of 7,000 synapses (connections to other neurons). All our negative thoughts and experiences get stored as memories. Every time we recall a memory, the synapses are strengthened. The more often these memories are accessed, the quicker and easier it is for negative thoughts to reappear (Crawford, n.d.).

Can the Brain Really Be Biased?

Negativity bias goes back to our ancestors and their need to be cautious of danger in the environment. Their survival depended on it. Of course, we have come a long way since we were cavemen hunting or being hunted. There is no need for us to be constantly on the lookout for danger, but this is an automatic process that starts to develop as infants and for some of us, the process is heightened to such an extent that negativity consumes us.

This negativity bias has been studied by psychologists for years. John Cacioppo, Ph.D., from the University of Chicago, studied electrical activity in the brain's cerebral cortex. Participants in his study were shown images that stimulated positive emotions and others that stimulated negative emotions. The negative stimuli caused a greater surge in electrical activity than the positive stimuli.

Neuropsychologist Rick Hanson, Ph.D., confirmed that the amygdala (the area of the brain that controls our emotions and motivation) uses approximately two-thirds of its neurons to detect negativity.

This means that two-thirds of your emotions and motivation are focused on the negative—the very definition of bias!

What's more, the amygdala then takes these super-charged, dominant negative neurons and very quickly stores them in the long-term memory. This is why we tend to remember negative or traumatic experiences more than positive ones. Why it's easier to remember an insult than a compliment. And why we think negatively more often than we do positively.

Cacioppo's research also found that we are more likely to make decisions based on negative information than we are positive information. Furthermore, negativity has a greater impact on our motivation. If you set goals, there is a greater chance that you will focus on what you will have to give up to achieve the goal instead of what you will gain from reaching it. (Cacioppo et al., 2014).

Imagine you have an argument with your friend or your partner. Even if the argument has been resolved, do you focus on the negative memories, experiences, and qualities or do you think back to all the good times you have had and why you love them? The brain is wired to think about the negative.

Why Do People Ruminate?

There is a difference between overthinking and ruminating. When we overthink, we are spending more time than necessary thinking about an emotion, action, or experience. A woman choosing her wedding dress is probably going to overthink because it is such an important decision. The decision isn't surrounded by negativity. Rumination is the act of overthinking about negative feelings, things that have occurred, or things that may or may not occur. Examples of rumination include the continuous thinking about:

- A night out when you drank too much and did something stupid

- A mistake you made during a presentation

- Failing an exam

- Having an argument with a loved one

- The fear of getting ill

- The fear of losing your job/a friend/a partner

- Global warming and the world coming to an end

- An upcoming social event where you will have to talk to strangers

- What if… and if only…

The list is endless because it very much depends on the individual. Some people may laugh at those who ruminate on the state of the planet, perhaps call them dramatic. But others might consider someone to be dramatic for worrying about things that are now in the past.

While talking to clients from all backgrounds with varying degrees of negative thinking, I put together a list of the most common, harmful negative thoughts that we ruminate over:

- I will never be able to do that

- They are better than me

- I failed/I'm a failure

- I will never forgive them

- I should have done something differently

- It's too late

- This is going to be a disaster

- It's far too difficult

- It ruined my whole day

One of the most common causes of rumination is that we feel like we are doing something about a problem. If you fear losing your job and live every day on eggshells expecting it to be your last day in the office, rumination takes over your mind. Our subconscious feels that by thinking about this problem, replaying different scenarios, we are seeking answers to prevent job loss. The initial fear of losing your job is replaced by what our mind believes is proactive problem-solving.

It's easy coming from someone who has such an enlightened state of mind. For the average human, rumination and worrying is not something that we can simply switch off. While everyone is going to worry about things at some point in their lives, when the worrying becomes problematic, i.e., it affects their work and relationships, it can develop into generalized anxiety disorder (GAD). GAD affects 6.8 million adults in the U.S. What is more concerning is that 25.1% of children between 13 and 18 are also affected by anxiety disorders (ADAA, n.d.).

Put It into Practice

A quick exercise for you. Think back to last week or last month and list 10 things you had worried would occur this week or this month. Now think about how many of them actually occurred. I will take a typical list of what I would worry about.

I was going to oversleep **X**

I was going to make a mistake with a new client **X**

I wouldn't be able to make it through my gym class **X**

The metro would crash **X**

My parents were going to nag me about spending time with them ✓

My parents were going to get sick **X**

I wouldn't have enough money to save toward my holiday **X**

My friends were going to laugh at my haircut **X**

My boss was going to fire me **X**

I was going to burn the dinner for friends that weekend **X**

One of my 10 worries came true and even this one was pretty much out of my control. This is in line with data on the validity of our worries.

According to researchers at the Pennsylvania State University, 91.4% of worries didn't come true for GAD sufferers (La Freniere & Newman, 2018). Which links back to negativity bias. Our brains are trained to think the worst and despite our logical intelligence, this natural occurrence is hard to stop.

Mistakes People Make When Dealing with Negative Thoughts

Again, when we look at mistakes we have made with our negative thoughts, it's not another reason to feel bad about ourselves. What has happened has happened and we can't change that. Being aware of common mistakes helps us to avoid making them in the future. If you read this while nodding your head, you can know that you aren't alone.

1) You see things in black and white

It's not always one or the other, right or wrong, happy or sad, good or bad. Life is far too messy to see things in just black and white. Rather than labeling something as either positive or negative, we need to see things as just what they are. When focused on one extreme or the other, we miss out on a wide range in between; this gray area can help us to see things in a different light and make better decisions.

It's also easier to make small changes when you stop seeing only black and white. Today you are feeling negative. There are a lot of steps in between negative and positive. To aim to be positive tomorrow might be a huge step that is just too big.

Instead, tomorrow, we need to aim to be OK; the next day, good; the following happy; and so on.

2) You brush your negativity under the rug

Out of sight out of mind! But this isn't the case with our negative thoughts. You might be able to push them to one side, but this won't resolve the problem. Ignoring the problem or pretending it doesn't exist can make it worse.

3) You tell yourself that things are out of your control

In many cases, this might be true. We have certainly seen how quickly control can be taken away from us over the last 18 months. The pandemic has taken people from us, cost us our jobs, even our homes, and for a long time, our freedom. Feeling like you are out of control is scary, but you have to remember there is always one thing that you can control: how you react.

4) You assume and make incorrect predictions

When thinking about what could happen, we tap into our memories to look for past experiences. If someone eats shellfish and gets food poisoning, they will recall this memory before eating shellfish again. If you go horseback riding and fall off, before going riding again, you are going to wonder if the same thing is going to happen. There is no evidence to suggest history will repeat itself. But because our negative memories are so predominant, topped with the tendency to think negatively, we will fall into the habit of predicting incorrect outcomes.

5) You see negativity only as negative

This is a good one, but have you ever thought about how negativity and anxiety work in your favor? You assume that you are going to miss your flight, so you create a backup plan. Walking home alone makes you anxious, so you take a cab, which is safer.

I'm not saying that we should celebrate the negative thoughts we have because there has to be a limit. It is important to realize that we also don't want a life that is 100% positive and that, like our ancestors, our anxiety and negativity can keep us a little bit cautious.

6) Your focus is on overcoming negativity rather than improving selfcare

Negative thinking is interlinked with multiple other issues. Our confidence is rock-bottom; we don't like who we see in the mirror or don't even recognize who we are. You're constantly stressed and tired. While we want to reduce the amount of time we spend ruminating, we also need to start looking after ourselves in a way we deserve.

Generally speaking, negativity is breeding and spreading like never before. This is thanks to the news, internet, and social media. When the Black Death began in Europe in October 1347, news of its deadliness wouldn't have reached the Americas. And it wouldn't have been on the news 24 hours a day.

In fact, thanks to the Olympics, we have recently had some inspiring international stories. But even then, there are people determined to spread negativity. We miss the days when social media was used to be sociable rather than feed the fears and hatred of others.

It's not all doom and gloom. If you look hard enough, you can see people in the world trying to make a difference. Companies replanting trees, countries welcoming those displaced by war, and the amusing images that do nothing except make us smile. Social media isn't all bad. Movements like #BlackLivesMatter and #MeToo enable global involvement to put an end to unjust behavior. It might be a negative haystack, but the positive needle is still there. The same is true for our negative thinking.

Just as scientists have spent a long time researching how the brain is wired and why we are prone to negativity, researchers are also looking at proven ways that we can overcome negative thinking patterns and even break the negative bias cycle. Some of the methods you might have tried before, and naturally, you are thinking that if they didn't work before, they aren't going to work this time.

Not every method works for everyone, which is why we are going to go over 7 simple steps, but each step will have various strategies to match different personalities. Even if you have tried strategies before, try again with an open mind. It might be that the first time you weren't mentally prepared, or you hadn't fully understood the root cause of your negative thinking.

Now that we have a solid understanding of negativity and rumination, and that our brains are wired in this particular way, we can begin to look at different thought patterns and clearly define where our negative thinking is stemming from.

Why Do I Worry So Much?

If you feel like you spend all of your time worrying over one thing or another, you are far from alone. Worrying is one of the most pervasive forms of negative thinking. We live in an age of instant information and constant communication, and while that brings with it a plethora of benefits, it can also make us very aware of just how much can go wrong in the world. From our health to the economy, from the state of our relationships to social injustice and climate change, we can find enough worries to occupy every waking second if we let ourselves.

Harmful vs. Normal Worry

A certain amount of worry is normal. Everyone experiences worried thoughts in stressful situations, such as when you're waiting on test results from your doctor or when a dip in the stock market hurts your retirement savings. Expecting to stop worrying altogether is unrealistic; if you put that kind of pressure on yourself, it could lead to even more negative thoughts and lower life satisfaction because you'll feel like you've "failed". Accepting that worrying is normal will help to take some of its power away.

Worrying can even be beneficial to your life in some cases, if it doesn't go to extremes. If you try to avoid worry by sticking your head in the sand and ignoring potentially dangerous or otherwise harmful situations, you won't be able to take steps to prevent them. For example, say your hours at work are being cut, which means your weekly take-home pay will be reduced. If you choose to ignore your worries about your new financial situation, you might not change your spending habits; you could end up going into debt or dipping into your savings unnecessarily. By allowing yourself to feel these realistic worries, however, you will be able to take steps to prevent financial duress. You might look into picking up part-time work or cutting back on more frivolous expenses. In this case, worry can help you react to a situation appropriately.

People who experience a normal amount of worry might also take better care of their health. Some studies have found that when people are worried about potential health problems, such as cancer, they might take better preventive measures, such as getting regular health screenings (Blaszczak-Boxe, 2017). Worry can help us look at life realistically rather than through rose-colored glasses. It allows us to be aware of potential dangers and ultimately navigate life more successfully. In other words, worrying is not necessarily negative in and of itself.

So, when does worrying cross over into problematic negative thinking? If you find that a specific concern is playing on repeat in your head for days or even months at a time, even though there is little evidence that it's something you actually need to worry about, that's a sign that your worrying has reached excessive, unhealthy levels. For example, worrying about your toddler falling down the stairs and deciding to install baby gates is realistic; worrying about media reports of mosquito-borne viruses in the next state over to the point of no longer letting your children play outside is excessive. Acknowledging realistic worries and then taking steps to resolve them is very different than replaying every potential negative outcome over and over again.

Similarly, if you are having difficulty making a decision about how to address or solve a problem in your life, your worrying might be standing in your way. Excessive worrying creates stress and strain in the body, and the natural human response to stress and perceived danger is the Flight, Fight, or Freeze reaction (Fight-Flight-Freeze, n.d.). Freezing up in the face of a decision is a sign that your worrying has reached excessive levels and is causing an unhealthy amount of stress.

Constant, excessive worrying also impacts your mental, emotional, and physical health. If you are having trouble falling or staying asleep because of repetitive worried thoughts or if you are sleeping more than normal in an attempt to escape from your stress, these are signs that your worrying has crossed over into a negative, harmful pattern. Worrying too much can also impact your cognitive function, making it hard for you to concentrate or remember details. If you find yourself feeling more irritable than usual or experiencing frequent headaches, jaw pain, or nausea and abdominal pain, these are all symptoms of excessive worrying. It's important to listen to your body's clues so that you can take steps to reduce your worrying, as long-term stress can lead to more serious health effects, including high blood pressure and ulcers. When you reach this point, worrying itself becomes the enemy that needs to be faced, rather than whatever problem you have been focused on.

In the next section, we'll discuss several ways to help you stop your worries from getting out of control.

How Can I Stop Worrying?

If left unchecked, your worries will feed on themselves and only grow stronger with time. For example, say you have a large deadline at work that is coming up very quickly. If you are overly worried about meeting this deadline, you might find yourself unable to concentrate on the work itself. Thoughts like, "I'll never get this done. Why didn't I start sooner? There isn't enough time in the day" begin racing through your head, distracting you and causing your worry to gain momentum like a runaway train. The more time and energy you spend worrying about not meeting your deadline, the further away from meeting it you actually get. This is the cycle of worry.

Take another example: your health. Perhaps you are concerned about some physical symptoms you've been experiencing. Instead of motivating you to go see a doctor, your worry might drive you instead to avoid getting medical attention so as not to receive bad news. While in the short term, it might make you feel better to not receive the frightening diagnosis you fear, in the long term, your concerns will just grow as your symptoms persist. In fact, you could end up facing an even worse diagnosis because you did not get help soon enough. In this case, your worry led to avoidance which in the end just gives you more to worry about.

One of the drivers of this cycle of worry is the amygdalae, two small, almond-shaped sections of our brain's temporal lobe. These areas of the brain are responsible for a range of survival instincts, including hunger, sex drive, and the fight-flight-freeze response mentioned earlier. When our bodies are under chronic stress, such as that produced by excessive worrying, it can send our amygdalae into overdrive. This results in heightened feelings of fear, anxiety, and worry. In addition, chronic stress reduces the ability of other regions of our brain, namely the hippocampus and medial prefrontal cortex, to rein in the emotional responses caused by overstimulation of our amygdalae (Ressler, 2010). If our amygdalae have become overactive due to stress and worrying, we can overestimate the actual level of risk or danger faced in a given situation. We will find even more to fear and worry about, thus creating further stress and further overstimulation of this area of the brain.

Question Your Worries

It can be difficult to stop the runaway train of your worries, particularly if worrying is a lifelong habit. The first step in stopping a negative thought pattern like excessive worrying is awareness. Once you have realized that you are worrying too much, you can adopt some simple strategies to help combat the habit.

One simple way to begin to slow down your racing thoughts is to question them. Next time you find yourself carried away by worry, simply take a few deep breaths and ask yourself the following set of questions:

- Is this worry rational or am I engaging in worst case scenario thinking?

- Is this worry something I can solve?

Questioning your worries helps in two ways. First, it acts like the emergency brake in that runaway train of thought, helping to stop it in its tracks. When you worry excessively, you have the same thread of thoughts, and sometimes even the exact same words or images, running through your head over and over again. By introducing a new thought like one of the above questions, you interrupt that repetitive stream. This helps to take away some of the worry's power because it is no longer dominating your mind. The simple act of ceasing to go down the rabbit hole of worry will likely give you immediate emotional relief.

Second, questioning your worries helps you to take action. When we are worried about an event or situation, we often feel helpless, like we are victims at the mercy of fate. Taking action, however small, can help us feel more in control and reduce our fearfulness. If we determine that our worry is rational, we can then decide how to proceed with addressing it. If it is irrational, however, we can choose to let it go; we can do this by using our intellect to point out the flaws in our own thinking and remind ourselves that there is in fact no reason for concern. Similarly, if we determine that our worry is solvable, we can then switch our focus to coming up with ways to solve it. If it is not solvable, we can choose to accept that reality rather than causing ourselves unnecessary stress about something we have no control over. We could instead choose to brainstorm ways to better deal with the uncertainty instead of just ruminating over the problem itself.

Let's take an example. Say you have a new boss who doesn't seem particularly friendly and who has been critical of your work in your last couple of meetings. You find yourself worrying constantly about whether or not your boss likes you; instead of simply doing the best job you can, you're consumed all day with trying to impress him and appear perfect. Your productivity and confidence start to go downhill. Soon you're walking into the office every day anticipating being fired and lying awake at night imagining losing your source of income and being evicted from your home.

We've all let such fear-based thinking run away with us on occasion. You can use the "question your worry" technique to break these fears down and examine them more closely. First, is your worry about your boss not liking you rational? Perhaps it is, but perhaps your new boss is just not overly friendly or demonstrative. More to the point, does it matter whether your boss likes you on a personal level? Plenty of colleagues work together successfully without necessarily having warm personal feelings for one another. What about your worry about getting fired? While your boss has given your work a series of critiques, that is also part of his job. It may not necessarily mean that he is unhappy with your work overall. What about your midnight worries over losing your source of income and ending up homeless? While tragedies do happen, this is clearly the worst case scenario and probably not particularly likely; you can write that particular realm of thought off as fairly irrational and not worthy of your attention at this point.

Now move on to the next question. Of the two fears you identified as at least somewhat rational—that your boss doesn't like you and that he's unhappy with your work and getting ready to fire you—are either of them solvable? If your boss truly does not like you, there is not much you can do about that other than continue to be friendly and professional and hope that he changes his mind with time. We cannot control other people's feelings, so trying too hard to solve this particular worry would be a waste of your energy. What about your worry that he is unhappy with your work? Now this is a problem you can take steps to solve. Make an effort to refocus at work and regain your lost productivity. Be sure to integrate the critiques he's given you into your projects. Perhaps set up a one-on-one meeting with him to discuss his expectations for you and to come up with a list of priorities for you to work on. All of these actions will not only likely make your boss more satisfied with your performance, they'll also make you feel more in control of the situation and less fearful.

The "question your worries" technique can help you see your worried thoughts with more clarity and more objectivity. You can go through this technique in your head or for even more powerful results, write it out in a journal or notebook. That way you can return to it when you feel those old worries beginning to pop up again.

Remember Past Successes

If disappointments have been flooding your mind, then it's only fair you remember past successes, however big or small they are.

When we're lost in constant worrying, it can be hard to believe that what we're fearing won't come to pass or that things will ever work out in our favor. It's easy to get sucked into all-or-nothing thinking at this point and tell ourselves that we'll never be able to accomplish a goal. A simple trick to cutting through these all-or-nothing worries is to bring to mind instances when you succeeded at something or when a situation did go your way. For example, if you're worried about a presentation at work or a test at school, recall a time when you aced a test or gave a perfect sales pitch. This will help to stop the cycle of worry by proving that things do indeed sometimes go well for you and that you have proven yourself to be perfectly capable of accomplishing goals. Recalling your past successes will also give you a much-needed self-esteem boost!

Put Worry on Your Schedule

According to a 2011 study, you might be able to reduce your worrying overall by setting aside specific windows of time in which you allow yourself to worry freely (Brownstein, 2011). Participants in the study were instructed to schedule 30 minutes a day during which they could think about their problems and brainstorm solutions; for the rest of the day, they were instructed to consciously avoid focusing on their worries as much as possible. The idea behind the study is that while telling people to stop worrying altogether is unrealistic, asking people to simply postpone their worrying until a more opportune time can be an effective way to break a pattern of constant worry.

Participants who set aside "worry time" experienced reduced stress and higher rates of success in treatment for anxiety disorders and other mental health issues (Brownstein, 2011). Putting worry on your schedule could ultimately help you worry less over time.

Reach Out for Help

Sometimes it can be hard to see our worries clearly. Our own fears loom large in our minds and often seem 100 percent justified to us. Getting an outside perspective can help us to see whether our worries truly are rational and solvable or whether we are giving in to worst case scenario or all-ornothing thinking. You can reach out to a trusted friend or family member to talk through your concerns. If you feel none of your loved ones are objective enough to help, there are various online and in-person support groups, as well as professionals like counselors, life coaches, and psychiatrists. Any one of these resources may be able to give you a fresh perspective on your worries.

Reaching out to other people can also open your eyes to potential solutions you may not have considered yourself. When we have run through a problem many times in our head, we can often have trouble thinking outside the box and coming up with new ideas. If you are dealing with a rational, solvable worry, a bit of crowd-sourcing might be just what you need to find the right solution.

Don't be afraid to reach out to people. It is good to know that you can rely on someone in your life.

Practice, Practice, Practice

Once again, your habit of excessive worrying did not develop overnight so fixing it will not be an overnight process either. It will take time to fully let go of a worry, particularly if it's one you've held for a long time. Do not beat yourself up when you find yourself getting caught up in worried thoughts. Simply return to the practices above without judgment and try again. With practice, your worries will gradually begin to loosen their grip on your mind and you'll experience longer and longer periods when you're not focusing on your problems.

As you go through this process, remember to celebrate your small successes as well. Any moment in which you can consciously choose to let go of a worry without following it down the rabbit hole is a step in the right direction. Take the time to pause and acknowledge your progress. If you feel comfortable with it, share your achievements with your loved ones or a therapist; their excitement for your success will give you even more motivation to keep going!

Eliminate Over Thinking

We have already discussed the difference between negative thoughts and rumination. While rumination may involve negative thoughts, it's more of a constant nagging feeling rather than a suffocating feeling.

Many people feel that ruminating leaves them spending too much time thinking about their past and future, a ditch that they are stuck in that prevents them from living in the present. There is no off button and people often find themselves up all night with these extremely intrusive thoughts.

In most cases, we are able to put some space between ourselves and rumination, but that doesn't stop the problem as we only beat ourselves up for overthinking and worrying.

We have to make an effort to stop rumination so that our pasts and futures don't define who we are in this moment. By doing so, we are able to live with more clarity and a better understanding of our circumstances.

Let's take a look at a real-life example of negative thinking and rumination.

Paul split up with his girlfriend about 6 months ago. She said some pretty harsh things about both his physical appearance and his personality.

His negative thinking caused him to replay these words over and over again. He believed he was a bad person and that his ex was completely right. He was a walkover, he had no backbone, and he had put on weight in their time together.

His rumination caused him to think about how he should have started playing football with his friends to control his weight. He thought about the future and how he was never going to have the confidence to meet another woman at his age.

He wanted to change his personality so that more people would like him. The changes he wanted to make overwhelmed him to the extent that he couldn't do anything about it.

Paul has to work on his negative thinking because the only thing his girlfriend had said that was based on evidence was the slight weight gain.

7 Ways to Combat Rumination and Overthinking

When rumination starts, you need to put a stop to it as quickly as possible. This way you can prevent it from spiraling out of control and leading to even darker thoughts.

As with many of our thought processes, the first step is to understand our triggers. What is it that has caused rumination to begin? Were you doing a particular activity or with a certain person?

Examples:

- Visiting a city you went to on holiday with your ex is going to stir up memories.

- Spending time with a toxic person may lead you to question how you aren't spending your time wisely.

- Cooking the same meals as your grandma who passed away will stir up feelings of loss and mourning.

- Watching a particular movie might bring up emotions related to your own experiences.

It's not to say that you won't ever be able to do these things again. It just means that before you revisit these triggers, you need to take control of your overthinking. Here is how!

1. Find a distraction

Many people find that rumination starts when the mind is at a loss for something to do. If you are focused on an activity, your mind is too busy to think of something else.

As soon as you spot the first signs of overthinking, get up and do something different. Go for a walk, do some cleaning, or read a book.

For these times, I highly recommend brain training apps and puzzles on your phone. Not only do you stop rumination, but you also give your brain a positive workout.

2. Talk to people

Sometimes, just a phone call to a friend or family member is enough to distract the brain. You don't need to discuss what is worrying you, especially if you are worried about how others feel about your constant worrying.

On the other hand, if you approach the subject in a way that doesn't come across as just complaining about your life, you can gain some amazing insights.

Rather than telling people what you are worrying about, let them know that you are worrying and ask for their advice on how you can overcome this.

People are much more inclined to lend you their ear when you want to do something about it instead of just complaining. You don't necessarily need to take their advice, but definitely consider it.

3. Make a plan

Rumination is often a trick our brain plays on us to think we are coming up with solutions when really, we are just stuck.

Define the problem that is causing your worrying in one sentence. Then start working backward through each step so that you have an actionable plan to resolve the issue.

Don't forget that each step must be small and manageable.

4. Don't wait to take action

I always advise people to make the first step on their action plan something that they can do straight away. If your plan begins with "talk to X about Y," you will do this the next time you see them. It gets the ball rolling.

If you are worried about your health and want to start eating more fruits and vegetables, don't wait till the shops are open. The first step of your action plan should be to find 3 new healthy recipes, which you can do straight away.

5. Question your overthinking

Just like with our negative thoughts, it's essential to decide if the cause of your rumination is justifiable.

Do you genuinely have a problem that you can solve or is the source of your worrying in someone else's hands? Are you losing sleep over a presentation, but your coworker is preparing the materials and you only have to show up? Is it possible that you have lost perspective and a molehill has now become a mountain?

Question your thoughts and challenge them.

6. Reassess your goals

Having goals is an important help to achieve our desires. Without goals it's easy to remain in this ditch with no movement. Sometimes, we set unachievable goals, and this causes us to dwell on how we are going to reach them instead of creating the plan to get there. We also have to be careful that our goals don't require perfectionism.

Isn't it better to first learn how to restore furniture and then work on perfecting your technique? Shouldn't you aim to run a half-marathon before a marathon? You can perfect a skill, with time. But if your goal is to get it perfect the first time, the act of starting will be even more daunting.

7. Give your self-esteem a boost

People who think poorly of themselves are more inclined to ruminate. Both rumination and low self-esteem can be linked to a greater risk of depression.

We are all good at something when we look hard enough. It can be something small like finishing a crossword in record time, bringing plants back from the dead, or cooking restaurant-quality desserts.

Don't feel you have to show your skills off to the world, but take time to enjoy these activities and build on them as well as learning new skills.

Next, we will take a closer look at some different types of rumination and how to overcome them, starting with how we can stop the past from interrupting our present and falsely predicting our future.

Learning How to Not Let the Past and Future Dictate Your Present

According to a study by psychologists Matthew Killingsworth and Daniel Gilbert, we spend 46.9% of our waking day thinking about something other than the task we are doing. That's nearly 47% of our time thinking about the past, the future, or events that may not even happen.

Our days are full of events, some appear meaningless and mundane like driving to work. Others are once-in-a-lifetime opportunities, creating memories with our children, parents, or friends. When we are unable to enjoy the present, our mind takes over and robs us of these special moments.

True, driving to work isn't exactly special, but we could find a way to enjoy it rather than overthinking. Why is it that we take time to create a delicious meal, but then eat it in a matter of minutes because there are other things to do?

We are stealing these small joys in life by worrying about what has happened or what is to come.

Like all types of overthinking, you want to knock this one on the head as soon as you realize your mind has started to think about the past. Do this by changing your activity to jolt your brain into a different thought.

We aren't going to just ignore the thought because it will keep coming back. We are going to schedule a time to deal with it.

When you are in the right frame of mind, often after exercising or achieving a small goal, readdress the past thought. To start with, you are now in control because it's not an automatic thought that has just popped up.

Rewrite the past event but with a more balanced and objective ending. You aren't going to change the result, but this will give you an opportunity to see both the good and the bad.

Imagine you had an argument with your parents, and you are still replaying what was said on both sides. Currently, you are still angry and upset and this might be influencing the way you are thinking and that it is all bad.

However, even though you could have phrased things in a more constructive way, you still managed to tell your parents the things they needed to hear.

Looking at it from a new perspective, you might see that while you should apologize for the way you spoke, you have a chance to reiterate what had been annoying you. The end result will be another conversation with your parents and a stronger relationship.

This is what we have characterized as mind-reading or fortune-telling. Regardless of what is most likely to happen, negative bias and past experiences cause our minds to jump straight to the worst-case scenario.

The absolute classic example of this is "We need to talk!" If it's your partner, you're getting dumped. If it's your child, they are dropping out of school. If it's your parents, they are dying. If it's your boss, you're getting fired. No one has ever heard the words "We need to talk" and thought they were getting a pay raise! The brain just isn't wired that way.

Still, this constant fear of what is going to happen in the future, known as anticipatory anxiety, can prevent us from concentrating. It can also impact our emotions and our ability to manage them. Physically, we can get jumpy or experience tension in our bodies. If this goes on for a long period of time, it's normal to have problems eating, sleeping, and going about our daily lives.

Anticipatory anxiety can be a symptom of social anxiety, phobias, PTSD, and panic disorders. In these cases, you might need professional help to get to the source of the anxiety, especially if it has developed into a fear that stops you from doing things (i.e., a fear of dogs stops you from going to any park and the sight of a dog causes a panic attack).

The most important way to overcome rumination about the future is to take care of your physical self. The connection between the body and the mind is extremely powerful and having a healthy body eases the strain on the mind. Creating a routine that includes a balanced diet, exercise, and enough time to get the necessary sleep is a great start.

You can also cut down on caffeine and sugar that tends to make people a little jittery. You can replace these habits with relaxation techniques to further relax the mind and body. There will be lots more on this later on!

They say never go to bed on a full stomach, but what is equally helpful is never to go to bed with a full mind! Bedtime is one of the worst times for rumination. There are no distractions and the silence seems to fuel our thinking.

Before looking at what you can do, take a moment to consider what you should avoid doing. As previously mentioned, caffeine isn't going to help you. Sadly, you should give up the afternoon coffee. For the best chances of falling asleep, you need to try and give up caffeine after 3 p.m.

Exercise is going to help but again, you need to choose the right time. Avoid aerobic exercise at least 90 minutes before you go to bed, or you will still be feeling the energy from the workout and it will impact your sleep cycle.

Be careful how late you work into the night. Today, it seems perfectly normal to be working at home in the evenings, even answering messages and emails up to the point of going to bed. You might feel like you are being productive and there is less to do in the morning, but the opposite occurs. If there isn't enough time between switching off from work and going to bed, you are going to take it with you.

You may also think that taking your phone to bed or watching a series on the tablet helps to distract your mind and makes it easier to fall asleep. Science tells us otherwise.

All electronic devices emit blue light. This blue light has a short wavelength, which delays the production of melatonin, the hormone that makes us feel sleepy. Not only do you want to avoid technology in the bedroom, but you should also look at changing bright light bulbs to warm colors that are more relaxing.

Creating a perfect routine to eliminate nighttime rumination

The perfect bedtime routine is going to vary from person to person. If possible, try to incorporate as many of these ideas as possible.

- Set a shut-off time for work. Ideally, this will be at least an hour be foregoing to bed. It will be hard to stick to this new rule at first but once you start getting more sleep, you will have more energy to achieve more throughout the day and it will be easier to say no to late-night jobs.

- Write your to-do list for the following day. Oftentimes, our brains go overall that we have to do the next day, worried about what we are forgetting. Take 10 minutes to seriously think about what needs to be done the next day and list these things in order of priority. Walk away and do another activity and then revisit your list in case there is anything missing. After a second check, leave it for the next day.

- Write in your journal. Like brain dumping the to-do list, writing in your journal gives you a chance to process thoughts and concerns rather than taking them to bed with you. End your journal entry with a few things that you are grateful for or some positive statements.

- Do something that is relaxing and makes you feel good. This could be meditation, having a warm drink, or a relaxing bath or shower. This can be 10 to 20 minutes of time just for you, a treat that you deserve after a long day. This can include face masks, preparing the next day's smoothie, or listening to your favorite vinyl—just a little time for self-care.

- When in bed, begin with progressive muscle relaxation. Tense your toes, breathe in, and hold for 5 seconds. Slowly exhale as you release the tension. Next, do the same for your calf muscles, and then your thighs. Work your way up until all of the tension is released.

- Read a book. A mattress review site asked 1,000 people about their sleep routine. Those who read slept for an average of 1 hour and 37 minutes more than those who didn't. Reading is an all-around healthy habit that can reduce stress, encourage empathy, and expand your vocabulary.

- Certain essential oils have been proven to promote a good night's sleep.

Lavender calms the nervous system. The combination of bergamot and sandalwood improved the quality of sleep in 64% of participants in one study (Dyer et al., 2016). Clary sage oil reduces cortisol levels, which negatively impact our sleep cycles (Lee et al., 2014).

- Finally, if you can't fall asleep and you find worrying thoughts stirring, repeat another round of progressive muscle relaxation and pick your book up again. If this doesn't have the right effect, get up before overthinking takes over. Take 20 minutes to do another activity before trying to go back to bed. This activity should be boring so that you aren't rewarding your brain. Try folding laundry or cleaning the toilet!

Don't give up on your bedtime routine. It can take anywhere from 18 to 254 days for a new routine to become a habit (European Journal of Social Psychology, 2009).

That doesn't mean it will take this long to see the benefits. And you may want to adjust small parts of your routine so that it is more effective. It's not an overnight fix but instead small, effective steps that will last a lifetime.

Coping with Unwanted Intrusive Thoughts

Intrusive thoughts are a type of negative thought. They are involuntary patterns of images or thoughts that are upsetting and may lead to depression. The images and thoughts are so strong that people can become obsessed with them. Intrusive thoughts are closely linked to OCD and substance abuse.

Intrusive thoughts are very much a part of everyday life. A study by Concordia University found that 94% of people experience these thoughts. We do, however, need to take control of these types of thoughts before they manifest into obsessive thoughts or more severe mental health problems.

Intrusive thoughts can be things like a fear that you are going to catch an illness or disease, which has been extremely common since the coronavirus outbreak. They might be images of breaking the law, hurting someone, or inappropriate thoughts or images of sex.

A married person might think about having an affair, a flash of an image if they see someone they have a crush on. When they can't get this thought out of their mind and it starts affecting their relationship, it has become an obsessive thought and possibly an underlying sign of OCD.

When somebody is suffering from intrusive thoughts of OCD, the fear will be very specific to them. Most of us at some point have worried about coronavirus, but only intrusive thoughts of OCD would focus on a specific fear like being killed in a car accident or a family member dying. The emotional distress this person feels can be indescribable, especially when they are so detailed. OCD intrusive thoughts can develop into severe social anxiety.

Like negative thinking and rumination, intrusive thoughts can be linked to depression. Furthermore, more than 25% of patients with OCD meet the criteria for a substance abuse disorder (Journal of Anxiety Disorders, 2008).

If you feel like your intrusive thoughts are out of control and they have developed into a more serious condition, it's a good idea to get professional help. Cognitive-behavioral therapy has been very successful in the treatment of obsessive thoughts.

How to conquer intrusive thoughts

1. Gain clear insight into your core values

The first step is to understand why these intrusive thoughts are causing you so much upset. The reason might be a trigger.

Unfortunately, if someone near your coughs one of the first images that springs to mind is that they have COVID-19, and you are now infected. Is this a reasonable intrusive thought?

There are numerous reasons for someone to cough, you may also be wearing a mask and have your vaccinations. Taking a practical approach helps you to determine whether the trigger warrants the thought.

For those thoughts that blindside you and don't seem to come from a logical occurrence, consider whether they go against your values.

An image of you hurting another human might be strongly against your beliefs, which is why it upsets you so much. For a sociopathic serial killer, the image isn't going to have the same impact. When you can clearly define your core values, you will understand why these thoughts cause such a strong reaction.

2. Let these thoughts pass through you

We can't block them or avoid them. Pretending they don't exist may cause you mind to give the thoughts more attention and this will be harder for you to overcome. To minimize the effect of the intrusive thought, accept it, acknowledge it, and visualize the thought passing through you as you move on.

3. Try not to react to fear or with fear

Although difficult, it's essential that you remember that this is only a thought and what you think or imagine is not a reality. If you imagine yourself as poor and homeless, it doesn't mean that you are or you are destined to be. We can feel an immense amount of fear from our intrusive thoughts, but we can't let the fear control us so that we end up doing something that isn't sensible.

Recognize that just because this thought has appeared doesn't mean that you have to act on it. Take a moment for some slow, deep breaths and with every breath, exhale that fear while the tension is released from your body.

4. Don't take your intrusive thoughts to heart

These are not messages from your subconscious describing your underlying desires. They are thoughts that you cannot control and do not make you a bad person. Feeling bad or even guilty about something that isn't reality and hasn't happened is only going to add to the mental strain.

Remind yourself how easy it is to let go of positive thoughts. You imagine you are going to win the lottery; you tell yourself it's not going to happen and move on without further emotions. Practice this with intrusive thoughts.

5. Don't change your life based on your thoughts

I have seen people avoid airports because of frightening images, parties because they fear they will make a fool of themselves, even driving a car because of thoughts of hitting a pedestrian.

People that change the way they live based on their intrusive thoughts aren't going to stop the thoughts. It just leads to living a life based on fears, which is heartbreaking as you can miss out on so much. Deal with the intrusive thoughts head on rather than trying to adjust your reality.

How to Stop Taking Other's Opinions to Heart

The worst advice I have heard time and time again is "Don't take things so personally." That's a wonderful idea but where is the advice? How do I actually do this? Wouldn't it be great just to have a thicker layer of skin and let others' opinions bounce straight off you? For most of us, it isn't that easy and it's a huge cause for rumination.

Here is how other people's opinions cause us to overthink. If you hold the door open for someone and they don't thank you, it is disrespectful. Our mind leads us to think that we are not worthy of respect, which can ruminate into feelings of worthlessness. If people look at you as if you have no worth, perhaps this is true.

Albert Ellis, the father of Rational Emotive Behavior Therapy, would tell you that it isn't the action that causes your emotions, but how you interpret the action. This interpretation is based on our beliefs.

If your belief is that it is polite to hold a door open for others, then you will be upset when you aren't thanked. If you don't believe it is necessary to hold the door open for people, or recognize that not everyone shares your belief, the action won't trigger the same emotions. The same theory can be applied to pretty much all of our actions. Consider the following acts and how your beliefs may differ from someone else's:

- Sharing food, office supplies, information

- Returning missed calls

- Tidying up after yourself

- Family occasions

- Changing the radio station in someone else's car

- Drinking the last of the milk and not replacing it or apologizing

Your partner might find it a huge nag that you always want them to go to family meals. You may feel that they don't like your family or don't want to spend time with you.

From their point of view, they grew up in a broken home and family occasions cause them to think about a childhood they missed out on. Not everyone will share your belief and by understanding this, it becomes easier not to take their actions personally.

Remember that not everything a person says is directly aimed at you. A pet peeve of mine is people who have large cars but are unable to park them. If I happened to mention this to you and you have a big car, it doesn't mean I am criticizing your parking. It's easy to take general comments and turn them into a personal criticism.

Instead of taking these general comments to heart and then ruminating about it for the rest of the day, you can politely ask the person if the comment was aimed at you. Yes, this will mean overcoming a fear of being criticized, but what's the worst that can happen?

If the comment was aimed at you, you can decide whether it is justified or not. If it is justified, you can make an improvement.

If not, you can remind yourself that their opinion isn't based on facts but solely their opinion. It's just as likely that they say it wasn't about you, and the rumination is stopped in an instant.

Empathy is a great help here. We are stuck in our own minds and trying to overcome our own problems. People may snap at us, gossip about us, or even just flat out lie. You have to get good at being the bigger person and to do this, don't drink in their poisonous opinions but instead, understand that they might be struggling with their own demons.

They too probably have negative thoughts and fears, problems they are trying to get to the bottom of. It's not fair or right that they take it out on you, but their opinions may be a manifestation of their own problems. How you react may only fuel them into hurting you more.

Make Wise Decisions and Solve Problems Faster

A common complaint is that our rumination creates a fuzzy blur in our mind; there is no clarity to our thinking, and this has a detrimental effect on our decision-making abilities. It's tempting to envy those who are good at solving problems.

They seem confident in their abilities and life appears to be more straightforward without all of the doubts.

Decision making is a learned skill. Some are naturally better at it than others but that's not to say that you can't improve your abilities. It's not that you can't make a decision, the problem is that your over-thinking clouds your judgment and causes you to doubt yourself.

Don't tell yourself not to overthink a decision. Instead, we are going to learn how to think smarter so that we can make the right choice with confidence.

Let's say you have to make a decision between a digital presentation and a hard copy of your information. Everyone is going digital, it looks flashier and professional but you feel that a tangible copy of information that clients can take away with them will be more beneficial. Your colleagues convinced you to go with the digital presentation last time and the results weren't as your boss had hoped.

There is a lot riding on this decision, and you feel the pressure mounting up. To make any decision wisely, the first thing to do is remove emotions and focus on facts. If there isn't data supporting an option, then it is an emotion. It's not to say that there isn't room for emotions in decision making, but they will cause you to ruminate.

Take yourself out of the situation and view the problem as an outsider. In this case, you could see things from your boss's point of view or the client's. What would be the most beneficial solution for them? Why are your colleagues so dead set against the idea? Is it because it involves more preparation? If so, how can you overcome this?

Solid decisions are made based on knowledge. Before even weighing the pros and cons of each possible outcome, ask yourself if you have sufficient knowledge. Knowledge can come from a wide range of sources. You might find that research on your clients tells you more about their likes, dislikes, and values.

Being assertive with your colleagues gives you a chance to listen to their thoughts and ideas, opening up new perspectives. Asking your boss for feedback on the last presentation highlights mistakes that were made and areas for improvement.

Finally, take a pen and paper and write down the potential outcomes of each of your options. Look at the worst- and best-case scenarios for each. Once you have weighed the options, which has more pros and cons?

Always set a deadline for decision making. If you really can't see a clear option, play the 1,2,3 game. No prior thinking and no delay in your response. Count 1,2,3 and say the first option that comes to mind. This works better when someone else is counting and you aren't expecting it, and your answer must be said aloud. Though you are lacking in confidence, it doesn't mean your gut instincts are wrong. The 1,2,3 game gives your intuition a chance to shine.

Put It into Practice

I know there are already many ideas that can help you to eliminate rumination but there is one final idea that I find fascinating and the studies prove its effectiveness. Self-distancing, and more specifically, the Batman Effect, are methods we can use to put distance between ourselves and our problems or challenges. This distance enables us to see things from a different perspective.

Self-distancing is the practice of thinking in the second person or using your own name. Rather than saying "I wish I could work harder" you would say "You wish you could work harder" or "Your name wishes they could work harder." When we use pronouns other than I, it has a similar effect to giving advice to a friend.

Many successful people, such as Beyoncé and Adele, have alternate personalities that they have created. When they imagine themselves as these people, they are better able to cope with nervousness and stress.

Researchers at the University of Minnesota (2016) asked children aged 4 to 6 to work on a repetitive task for 10 minutes. They had the option to take breaks if they wanted. The children were asked to repeat one of the three following questions as they worked:

- Am I hardworking?

- Is (their name) hardworking?

- Is (their favorite character, i.e., Batman, Dora the Explorer) hardworking?

Those who used their name performed better than those who used the first person. But it was those who imagined themselves as their favorite character that took fewer breaks, worked harder, and enjoyed the activity more. In fact, these children spent 23% more time on the task at hand compared with the children thinking in the third person.

The next time rumination rears its head, try self-distancing or creating your own alternate persona so that you have a little more space to think about the situation in a different, and often more rational, way.

Up to now, we have spent the majority of the time focusing on strategies to beat negative thinking and rumination. You now have a massive range of tips and tricks, backed by science. However, with the constraint strain and pressure we face today, high amounts of stress can quickly undo the work we have done.

How to Control Your Mind

Become the Conscious Observer of Your Thoughts

On a moment-to-moment basis, our thoughts tend to act like white noise or background music. They flow through our mind effortlessly without attracting much notice. They also do not hang around for too long; if left to their own devices, thoughts pass through our minds quickly. One minute, you're thinking about what to cook for dinner and then suddenly you find yourself reminiscing about something funny your spouse said that morning. Sometimes, though, we become attached to a particular thought and begin to follow it. That one thought leads to another related thought and another and soon you have lost an hour of your time following this train of thought. Sometimes this habit can be pleasant, like when you get lost in a fun daydream. If you become attached to a negative thought, though, you can quickly get sucked down a rabbit hole of negativity. This is when that one small snowball of a negative thought picks up speed and starts to become an avalanche.

There is no way to stop an avalanche once it has started. The only way to stop an avalanche is to prevent it from occurring in the first place. While it's not completely impossible to stop the spiral of negative thoughts, it's much easier to prevent that spiral from even starting. How do you do this?

Awareness

As we said before, you cannot change what you are not aware of. In order to stop following the path of random negative thoughts, in order to learn how to just let them pop into your mind and then pop back out again naturally, you first need to see your thoughts. You need to learn to observe your thoughts consciously, neutrally, and non-judgmentally.

Whenever you are presented with a situation, try and notice the way you react to it. Were you angry when the driver cut you off in front of you? Was the reason for your anger the driver or something bigger?

When you begin to evaluate your situation, you might notice that things are not as clear-cut as they seem.

Perform a Brain-Dump

When the garbage in your house begins to fill up, what do you do? You obviously empty the trash can. You don't want that pile spilling over!

Take the time to write down your thoughts to perform a brain dump.

It's the same with your brain. Not all the information you have in your brain might be useful to you. Or you might be feeling down about your personal life or work. Sometimes, it feels as though there is a hurricane going through your brain and you are unable to focus on a thought or add new thoughts to your brain. It might truly become overwhelming for you to think.

But why exactly does your brain become overwhelmed?

Think of your thoughts like the tabs of your internet browser. You have opened a few tabs because you deem them important. As more tasks get added to your life, you open even more tabs. However, you forget to close the old ones. Eventually, you have a hundred tabs open and you are shifting from one tab to another, trying to get a bearing on your thoughts.

In such cases, you perform a brain dump.

A brain dump is a process where you get the thoughts out of your head so that you can deal with them. The process helps you focus on one thought at a time and even prioritize them. So how do you do a brain dump?

Step 1: Get a Pen and Paper (Or You Can Use a Word Processor)

I recommend using a pen and paper because it gets your brain to focus on what you are writing. When your brain is focused, you are able to process information better.

Step 2: Make a List

Your next step is to write down every plan or activity that comes to your mind. Do you have a project you need to finish at work? Perhaps a birthday party that you need to attend? Did you make movie plans with someone? Whatever it is, write it down on a sheet of paper.

Step 3: Take a Walk

When you have finished listing as many things as you can remember, get up from your place and take a walk. Walk for about 5 to 10 minutes and then return to the sheet of paper. Focus on it again and you might remember some things that you hadn't thought of earlier. Add them to the list as well.

At this point, you might have a pretty big list in front of you.

Step 4: Categorize

Start categorizing your list into various sections. Here is an example that you can make use of:

- Personal

- Home

- Work

- Freelancing Stuff

- Projects

- Work Ideas

- Plans

- Errands

- Important Dates

You can create your own list based on your requirements. But make sure that you have a list that ties in with your requirements and goals.

Step 5: Break Down the Projects

Now take each task and break them into smaller objectives. Something as simple as "get a carton of milk on the way home" does not have to be broken down any further. But if you have a task such as "complete your work project by the end of the week," then find ways to break it down into manageable and achievable portions.

This step is not mandatory. So, if you think that you cannot break down any tasks, then don't force it.

Step 6: Add Schedules

In this step, you are going to prioritize your tasks. Look through the list and find out all the tasks that you can complete immediately. Then move on to the next set of tasks in order of priority. As you move down the list, make sure that you are giving a timeframe for those tasks that cannot be completed at a specific time.

Another way that you can split the tasks is by the below categories:

- Tasks that should be done today

- Tasks to complete within this week

- Tasks to complete within this month

- Things to do after this month

- Unimportant things

Anything that you place into the unimportant things category should be forgotten about since they don't matter. You should be critical about your list. Your list should ideally be concise so that you can sort through the important things. The main purpose of a brain dump is to filter out the unwanted ideas that flood your mind.

Step 7: Start Working

As soon as you have completed your list, focus on the task that you have to do immediately. The earlier you can start working, the faster you can get through the tasks.

The list can always increase in length. If you feel that you have more to add, then add them and follow the steps above to give them a timeframe or schedule.

Get Out of Your Head and into Your Body

It is tempting to entertain your thoughts. There is a need to solve them in your head. You brood over them thinking that you are going to find an answer to them only to realize that the only thing you managed to accomplish was a splitting headache.

Don't spend too much time on your thoughts. Rather, write down the problem on a piece of paper. Then use the steps below to deal with it.

Step 1: Identify the Problem

Write down the nature of the problem and other details that you can add to the list. For example, let us say that you are a graphic designer and you have to create 5 creative samples of an advertisement. Note down the problem by using the questions below:

- What do you have to do?

- Are there any specific requests?

- What should you avoid?

- What would you consider as a job well done?

- What do you think shows poor quality?

- Does the client have any objectives that they would like to focus on?

Add other questions that you feel are pertinent to gather more information about the task.

- Do you have any sources of information that you would like to refer to?

- Can you get any help solving the problem? It could be your friends or your colleagues.

- Do you think you can put in a request to your boss for assistance?

- Do you have samples that you can use to inspire you?

Whatever materials you have that can help you can be added to this section.

Step 3: Provide Solutions

Take your time to come up with as many solutions as you can for the problem. List down any creative ideas that you think can help you finish the tasks quicker. Make sure that you list down the details of the solution. Do not just keep bullet points of what you would like to do. You need to have a written record of what you would like to do in case you forget the solution in the future.

Step 4: Provide Alternatives

Let us assume that the worst comes to pass and you are unable to complete the tasks on time. What do you do then? Do you have an alternative strategy? Can you deal with any delays that might arise during the completion of the task? What would you do if you lost creative inspiration? Make sure that you have a list of all available alternatives to deal with a plethora of unexpected circumstances.

Step 5: Plan of Action

There is no point in making a plan if you have no actions to back it up. Your final step is to list down all the actions that you are going to take in order to complete the task at hand.

Make sure you give schedules and timeframes for the actions. Do not give too much wiggle room to complete the tasks. When you give your mind the chance to look for chances to delay your work or take long breaks, then rest assured, it usually does look for a way to ease things.

Now that you have a plan set for your project, there is another important question you might have to deal with; what happens if you cannot create a plan to deal with your problem or task?

In that case, you have nothing to worry about because events are beyond your control. You should focus on removing the worries you have about the problem out of your head and keep your attention focused on the things that you can handle in front of you. This might be tricky. You might be tempted to return to the problem. But unless you can deal with it, you shouldn't be thinking about it too much.

Become Emotionally Strong

Your mind can sometimes wander when it is faced with an emotional task. Emotions can also distract you from the things that are important, cause unwanted levels of stress, or even project unhealthy negativity into your mind.

While it is not wrong to show your emotional side, it is not right to let your emotions take control of your life too much. Being emotionally strong allows you to approach your life with tact and rational behavior.

But how can one become emotionally strong? Here are some ways to go about it.

Set Boundaries

Whether it is with your friends, family members, relatives, or even your colleagues, it is important that you set some boundaries for yourself. If you do this, you will understand where you stand in all matters of life. People won't take advantage of your kindness or treat your emotions as though they did not matter. They won't just start assuming that they can do anything to you. When you create a degree of tolerance and acceptance, then you are effectively laying down the foundation for emotional strength.

Forget the Past

Do not let the past become a ghost in your life, haunting you at every turn and reminding you of your failures, pain, disappointments, incapabilities, or weaknesses. Do not try to emotionally autopsy your past. Rather, try and learn from them. Figure out how you can use them to become a better person. In fact, the past does not exist. The flow of time cannot go backwards (despite what the science-fiction movies tell you). Your past is officially a thing only present in memories. Let it stay that way. Your only reason for thinking about them is to plan the future.

Ask for Help

Whether you simply need the company of your friends or a shoulder to cry on, reach out to someone. Having people listen to you not only lightens the burden, but also reminds you that you are not alone in this world. If you need help, don't be afraid to ask. Do not automatically label yourself as a burden. Even if people think you are a burden to them, do not think of yourself as such. You should be cutting ties with such people, as they have made their intentions clear. Do not surround yourself with toxic people, who only attach labels on you and are absent whenever you need them the most.

Discover the Joy of Your Company

You are the protagonist of your story. If you have watched the recent Avengers movie, then you might have a favorite character. It could be Iron Man or it could be Black Widow, but there are characters you love because they are cool, smart, confident, powerful, or for any other reason. In the same way, look at the things that make you seem awesome in your eyes. Why do you love you? What makes you special? What do you like to do?

As you discover more about yourself, you will have more reasons to enjoy your own company. Try to engage in your passions or activities that you enjoy doing.

Enjoy spending time by yourself.

Take Care of Your Body

The body is a temple; respect it and take care of it. Don't allow your health to deteriorate. Try and exercise as frequently as possible. Even brisk jogging will do. Eat a well-balanced meal. Make sure that you are keeping your body in peak condition. Avoid using substances such as nicotine, alcohol, and caffeine too much.

And while you are taking care of your body, make sure that you...

...Take Care of Your Mind

The mind is a powerful tool. And just like all tools, it can suffer wear and tear over time. Keep healthy mental habits so that you keep your mind fit. Try and meditate. Engage in mentally stimulating activities. Do not overload your mind and give yourself as much rest as possible.

And if you really have to, then go ahead and take a vacation. You probably deserve it.

In today's world, almost everything is documented on social media. People are tempted to get into discussions and spend their mental energy trying to win over random strangers on the internet. Remember to pick your battles. Do not start an argument with each and every person you meet online. At the same time, do not look to engage in an emotional argument with people in your life if you really don't have to. Does someone prefer something that you do not like? Let it go. Live and let live. Do you feel like people have different opinions on a particular subject? Then don't try too hard to bring them on your side.

Benefits of a Thoughts Journal

One of the ways to deal with overwhelming thoughts or emotions is to express them in healthy ways. Rather than break objects when you are angry or frustrated, you can instead choose to divert all that energy into something more rewarding.

This is where a journal becomes useful. When you use a journal, you:

- Are able to manage anxiety

- Can reduce stress effectively

- Can cope with depression

So how do you record your thoughts in a journal effectively? Here are a few tips that you can use:

Journal Tip #1: Try to Write Every day

Be consistent when you journal your thoughts and ideas. Ideally, you should be journaling your thoughts every day. If you feel that writing in a book is not efficient, then you can make use of the numerous journal software and applications that are available. This way, you don't have to worry about running out of pages. You do not need to spend an hour or so writing. Simply set aside a few minutes and describe your day. Talk about anything that you would like to express. If you feel that you had reacted negatively or experienced negative thoughts or emotions, then mention the reason for the negativity. Allow yourself to express freely. When you are done, go back and read your entry. Think about the situation and see if you can write down a possible solution for the outburst of negative thoughts or reaction. Don't worry if you cannot find a proper solution.

Journal Tip #2: Carry Your Journal with You

Try to keep your pen and paper or your journal application with you at all times. This way, you can create an entry any time you feel like it. Write down the entry when the thoughts are fresh in your memory so that you can express yourself better.

Journal Tip #3: You Don't Have to Be a Writer

The important rule of journal writing is this: write whatever feels right! Don't worry about how you sound. This is your journal and it should be used to express yourself freely. It is your private space to pen your thoughts and discuss the things that matter to you. Do not hold back the words. Sometimes, you might be surprised by the emotions behind your words. Do not be alarmed by it. Let the words flow through your hands freely. And you don't have to worry about what others think. After all, it is not like you are going to publish your journal!

Journal Tip #4: Your Journal, Your Rules

If you feel like you would like to share your journal with someone, but are not sure if it is the right thing to do, then try the following instead. Take a journal entry that you would like to talk about and then discuss that with your friends or family. See if you are comfortable communicating your thoughts to them. Then check if they are receptive to your thoughts and emotions. If you feel comfortable talking to them, then you can choose to share more of your journal entries.

The Power of Sleep

A good night's sleep is something we all crave to a point where we feel like the phrase "good night's sleep" is nothing but a myth.

The reality is that a good night's sleep is as important as a healthy diet and exercise. In fact, if you are working out, then one of the routines that you have to incorporate into your life is a good night's rest.

In today's fast-paced world, people are finding it difficult to get the required hours of sleep. At the same time, the quality of sleep has decreased as well. Let us see why sleep is important.

Weight Gain

Did you ever think that sleep could actually be connected to weight gain? Seems like a farfetched idea, doesn't it? In fact, one might claim that I am creating connections when none exist. Sadly, there does exist a link between poor sleep and weight gain, which has also been documented by a research (Cappuccio et al., 2008). Based on the results of the study, children and adults who do not get the recommended sleep hours are 55% to 85% more likely to become obese.

Good Sleep = Fewer Calories

When you get a good night's sleep, then your mind is active. It only requires the necessary amount of nutrition that you feed it on a daily basis. However, when you are sleep deprived, the body and mind require even more energy to function normally. Eventually, people start consuming more coffee and more sugar, just to get through the day. The body also increases the production of ghrelin, which is the hormone that triggers appetite in the body.

When you get a good night's sleep, then your body arranges the memories, thoughts, and ideas of the previous day. It does this so that when you wake up in the morning, it is as though your mind has a clean slate to start with. You are able to absorb memories better, which increases the brain's concentration levels, and eventually contributes to better productivity.

What happens if you are sleep deprived? Firstly, all those memories from the previous day won't be arranged and catalogued properly by your brain. You wake up with your head full of thoughts, which cause headaches in some people. Secondly, the brain cannot store more memories. It is like adding water to a cup that is already full. Your concentration then begins to diminish and you find yourself unable to store more information. When you can't take in new information, then you won't be able to take in the information that matters. For example, let's say that you have to manage an important business event for your company. You are in charge of everything, from finances to the logistics to marketing of the event. Since your brain is unable to take in more information, you begin to forget things easily. You might have taken into account a piece of information recently, but because of your memory, you won't be able to recollect it because your brain disperses the information. Your productivity lowers and that eventually starts showing in your work.

Getting Physical

Sleep also increases physical performance. With proper sleep, you feel well rested. It's like putting the battery of your mobile device to charge; after you disconnect the charger, you are going to have longer-lasting battery power. In fact, research conducted on poor sleep has shown that proper sleep has improved performances in basketball players (Mah, C. D., Mah, K. E., Kezirian, & Dement, 2011).

Glucose

Lack of sleep affects blood sugar levels and also decreases insulin sensitivity.

As you might know, insulin is a hormone produced by the body that creates glucose from carbohydrates from the food that you consume. The hormone keeps your blood sugar levels from becoming too high, a condition called hyperglycemia, or too low, known as hypoglycemia. When the sensitivity of insulin reduces, then it won't be able to detect the carbohydrates in the body. This might prevent it from getting the required amount of glucose into the body, which eventually leads to hypoglycemia.

Depression

The links between sleep and mental state is a complicated one. When you have improper sleep patterns, then your brain loses its mental strength. This brings about big shifts in your emotions. These emotional fluctuations are exhausting for the brain to deal with. Imagine this scenario playing out. You have spent a long day at work and you are exhausted beyond belief. All you can think of is just relaxing for a bit. However, you realize that you still have so many chores to take care of. You would not exactly be at your peak performance now, would you? Your brain goes through the same process. It is too exhausted to deal with the emotional fluctuations and just lets your mind feel the full brunt of all emotions it receives, good or bad. When all the negative emotions you feel are unfiltered, you officially have a recipe for poor mental health. All of the negative emotions eventually cause depression, stress, and even anxiety.

How to Get Proper Sleep?

There are a few tricks you can use to improve the quality of your sleep.

Increase Daylight Exposure

Your body has a natural method of keeping time known as the circadian rhythm. This rhythm is based on the different times of the day. It tells your hormones, body, and brain when to stay awake and when it is time to rest. Exposure to natural sunlight helps you maintain your circadian rhythm. Have you ever been in a situation where you have been spending so much time indoors that when you look outside the window or step outside, you are surprised that so much time has passed and it is already dark? If you find yourself in such situations, then you need to change your habits. Continually disrupting your circadian rhythm causes your body to keep you awake, thinking that it is not time for bed. Eventually, it is pushing past the limits of exhaustion and you are not aware of it. This causes insomnia and you end up feeling sleepy way later than you should, causing you to receive less sleep.

Get yourself some natural sunlight. Try and take breaks outside as much as possible in order to get your body used to the time of day.

Blue Light Exposure

Daylight improves sleep patterns. But what about lights at night?

Research has shown that nighttime light exposure, especially blue light, causes you to lose sleep (Fonken et al., 2010). Once again, this has got to do with your circadian rhythm. The blue light confuses the brain into thinking that it is still daytime. Your brain becomes instantly more alert. This is why many people stay on their mobile devices, going through their social media feed until late into the night. They claim that they use their phones because they are unable to sleep, little do they know that they are unable to sleep because they are using their phones. When people who are used to scrolling through their mobile devices late at night try to sleep early, it becomes a bit of a challenge for them.

Avoid Caffeine Late at Night

Caffeine increases focus and energy. Which is why having it late at night only makes you want to stay up late. The caffeine enters your nervous system and stimulates it, preventing your body from relaxing late at night.

Avoid Irregular Sleep Patterns

Your body will give you a signal to fall asleep at certain times of the day because it is used to the fact that you fall asleep at the same time every day. In fact, have you ever experienced a time where you automatically wake up in the morning without the help of your alarm? You often wonder if you are getting used to waking up at that particular time. The truth is; you are. When you stick to a schedule, the body automatically adjusts its internal clock to support your timings. But what happens when you keep disrupting this schedule? Well, in that case, your body simply starts giving you mixed signals. You start feeling tired when you are not supposed to, such as in the middle of your work.

Don't Consume Too Much Alcohol

Better yet, avoid alcohol altogether. Alcohol is known to increase the causes of sleep apnea (Issa & Sullivan, 1982).

Sleep apnea is a serious sleep disorder that is characterized by irregular breathing during sleep. As you drift off to sleep, your breathing stops and starts up again without any warning.

Because of this breathing pattern, you might not get a good night's sleep. This causes you to have poor sleep. When you wake up in the morning, you are left feeling drowsy and tired. Sleep apnea is even dangerous as you might wake up gasping for air. In other words, you are at a risk of suffocating while you sleep, which is a definitely frightening prospect.

Improve Bedroom Conditions

Is your bedroom too hot? Do you have too much light filtering through the curtains? Do you smell something odd or hear the sounds of dripping water from the kitchen? All of these sounds, sights, and smells distract your brain from focusing on sleep. Certain people are used to disturbances and have trained their brain to ignore them during sleep. But that only accounts for a small part of the population. Most people are not used to facing disturbances during sleep.

Your bedroom should be a place where you can relax. Try and optimize your bedroom settings. Remove any artificial light from electronic devices such as digital clocks, computers, and mobile devices. Make sure that your bedroom is a quiet and relaxed place for you to get a good night's sleep.

Clear Your Mind in the Evening

Try not to go to bed with your head filled with thoughts. If you want to, you can meditate for a while before you head to bed. You can also listen to relaxing music, take a warm bath, or read a book to encourage you to fall asleep. One particular method may not work for you so try experimenting until you find the best way to put yourself to sleep.

Check Up

You might not have any sleep disorders, but it is better to get expert advice on the matter. Head to your local doctor and see if you need to receive treatment for any sleep conditions. No one likes to be told that they have a sleep disorder. However, it is far better to know that there is something and get it treated than ignore it until it becomes worse.

Make Sure You Have a Comfortable Bed

Some people wonder why it is that they find it more comfortable to sleep in a hotel.

The reason is simple. Hotel beds are made for comfort. Make sure that you bring the same level of comfort to your bed as well. If you need two pillows, add them. Need a thick blanket? Get one. With proper sleeping conditions, you will avoid problems such as backaches, neck stiffness, numbness in various parts of the body, and other physical problems.

Exercise and Yoga

But not before bed! You do not want to pump your body full of adrenaline right before you catch some Zs. When you exercise, you are encouraging your body to get rid of all your muscle tension, relaxing them. The same goes for yoga as well. When you eventually fall asleep, your body is ready to relax.

Avoid Fluids

Do not drink too much fluid before going to bed. This causes nocturia, which is a condition where you feel compelled to urinate excessively during the night. This causes you to repeatedly wake up in the middle of the night, interrupting a good night's sleep. In some cases, people find it difficult to head back to sleep once they are woken up by nocturia.

Avoid drinking fluids at least 1 or 2 hours before you head to bed.

Bottom Line

If you find yourself getting less sleep than required, then try and evaluate your sleep patterns, conditions, and your health.

Check and see if the environment you are sleeping in is comfortable. If your sleeping patterns are irregular, then you can work on that. Check that you are eating a proper diet before heading to bed (try not to eat too close to bedtime) and that you are getting proper exercises during the day. Look through the solutions provided above and then see if any applies to your situation. And if you feel that you have tried everything and you still have difficulty sleeping, don't hesitate to visit the doctor. It's better to receive a proper solution to your problem.

Discovering New Good Habits

Habits are powerful. They are truly influential.

To understand their power, one has to delve deeper into the mind, where we discover who – or what – is truly in control.

Think about this situation. You are headed home from work or any other point of origin. What matters is that you have taken the route home multiple times in your life so you know it like the back of your hand. One evening, you are taking this route when you realize that you are supposed to stop by the supermarket to purchase a carton of milk. As you plan out the evening, thoughts of the milk move on to the time you tried that incredible milkshake with your friends. Ruminations of your friends make you ponder about your weekend plans. You think it might be a fun idea to catch a movie at the local theatre or play a round of pool. That just reminded you, isn't it your friend's birthday next month? Perhaps you should get him something. If only your boss would give you your yearly bonus. But boy, you have so many projects to get done Wait a minute.

You have already reached home. But how? You don't remember the entire journey.

What you have experienced is a phenomenon called "highway hypnosis," which is like the distant cousin of line hypnosis. Your subconscious mind took control over your movements while your conscious self focused on the thoughts zipping through your brain. When you eventually reach your destination, your subconscious mind recognizes it and gives back the control to your conscious mind.

Even now, your subconscious mind is performing so many calculations as you read the words on this page. Your breathing, posture, blinking, heart rate, the way you are sitting, and so many other parts of your position are controlled by the subconscious mind.

So, you see, the subconscious mind is truly influential. What makes it powerful is the fact that you are never aware of its influence. It's a mental nudge and suggestion that goes mostly unnoticed. Everything is automatic. The confident feeling you get when you are wearing a suit or dress? That's your subconscious mind taking cues from your brain and the environment to create a response. The reason you feel pangs of sympathy for the homeless on the street? It's your subconscious mind pushing those thoughts into your brain.

Don't believe me? Then think of the last time that you saw someone who was disabled, homeless, or suffered from a form of debilitation and felt like that you wanted to help them. Do you remember each and every thought process that went through your head and forced you to arrive at the emotions you were feeling? Did you plan the course your mind would take in order to make you feel something? It felt like the emotion was just there when you felt it, didn't it?

This is your subconscious mind influencing you. In fact, the majority of emotions that we feel are spontaneous and encouraged by our subconscious mind.

But doesn't that make you think? If the subconscious mind does influence our emotions in such ways, who gave the directions to our subconscious to react in such a manner toward that particular scenario? When a barista gets our order wrong, why does our subconscious mind compel us to feel annoyed rather than be kind and forgiving?

That is dependent entirely on you.

When you act in a particular way, the subconscious mind records your actions and creates a mental program out of it. This program is used as a template for future actions. Your subconscious mind does this because you cannot handle each and every stimuli or situation that plays out in front of you. It would overwhelm your senses and overload your brain. Hence, your subconscious mind takes some of the workload while you can focus on other, more important things.

This method used by the subconscious – where a stimulus from the past affects your actions, thoughts, or feelings in the present – is called priming. And priming is a powerful tool used by your subconscious mind.

For example, if you have been ignoring your alarm clock to get extra sleep, your subconscious mind records that activity. Now every time you hear the alarm clock, you are capable of switching it off and going back to sleep. Sometimes, your subconscious mind throws in thoughts and images of how comfortable sleep really is just to entice you to return to bed. In some cases, you might even sleep past the alarm!

And that's where your bad habits come from.

The more you prime your subconscious mind to focus on bad habits, the more it incorporates them into your life.

Have you ever noticed people wake up in the morning and read motivational quotes? What they are doing is priming their brains, even though they don't realize it. By teaching the brain some motivational quotes, they are giving it a set of priming instructions. When they experience a challenging moment during their day, the subconscious mind goes back to the prime, which in this case are the motivational quotes, and uses them to add motivation into people's lives. When you start keeping your home clean, you feel clean because your subconscious mind has learned about how cleaning is good.

The Habits

The Good Habits, The Bad Habits, and The Ugly Negativity

When you have good habits, you automatically start organizing your life, managing your time, and getting more focused.

You organize your life and make sure that things are in order in your house.

You ensure that you do not delay tasks or work. There are schedules placed for various tasks. In little ways, you start removing chaos so that order can be ushered in.

The more order you create, the more efficiently you use your time. For example, by waking up early in the morning, you realize that you do not want to simply waste time, for that would be a bad habit. Rather, you go through the day's schedule, organize everything, get some exercise, and prepare a healthy breakfast. One by one, you eliminate your bad habits until you have very few of them.

You focus better as well. Once you start eliminating bad habits, you don't have unwanted thoughts distracting you. Additionally, you have completed your tasks on time. You now have the time to focus on other important things.

Each good habit you cultivate continues to pile up and bring more order into your life. Your subconscious, now inundated with all of these good habits, is slowly shooting positive messages into your brain. You become a better person.

But how is all of this related to negative thinking?

Let's take the example of waking up early in the morning. Your alarm rings but you shut it off and promptly sink your head into the pillow again. You don't want to deal with the day and it seems like you are well on your way to getting some extra shut-eye. This act convinces your subconscious that you would rather sleep than be active. Anytime you feel mentally exhausted, rather than take a walk or relax for a bit, you automatically start thinking of sleep. Over time, you notice that your body starts to feel sluggish. You end up believing that you're not a morning person. Because you did not have a good start to your day, this attitude carries forward into the rest of the tasks that you perform throughout the day. When you start seeing how your life revolves around bad mornings, lazy routines, and poor performances, during the rest of the day, you start to develop a negative outlook on life. Add to the fact that you have allowed so this all to happen and you have a recipe for negativity.

This becomes a cycle. You begin to attract more negativity, which teaches your subconscious mind to develop an unhealthy outlook on how to deal with situations. You begin to express your negative thinking in your actions. If someone accidentally bumped into you, rather than accept their apology, you respond with a scowl that could send people running for their dear lives. In such ways, you become a negative person. And the worst part? You don't realize the changes happening to you. Everything feels natural as the subconscious mind does not make these changes obvious. If you had used your conscious mind to make changes, then you would have been aware of them. But since your subconscious mind is the guide here, you think that things are the way they are because that's who you are.

This normality is harmful because it is easy to get used to. Think about this; when being lazy is normal, then why would anyone fight it? To make things worse, we also have to consider the psychological phenomenon of hindsight bias.

In Hindsight

Have you ever been in a situation where someone was telling you something and you exclaimed, "I was just about to do that"

You see, the brain wonderfully stores information. And edits them as well.

When you are in a situation where someone else beats you to the chase, your brain does not want to make you feel incompetent or slow. And so, as soon as the other person reveals the solution, your brain takes in the information, plants it in your memory, and erases parts of your old memory where you did not know the solution. This way, you feel as though you knew the solution all along. This phenomenon is known as hindsight bias and it is not always a bad thing.

You see, when you have too much related information in your brain, they all vie for control and attention. This leads to confusion, a jumbled-up memory, and unreliable information in your brain. And so, your brain deletes old memories so that you won't accidentally remember them. This system allows you to draw on the most relevant or recent memories that you have.

But where hindsight becomes harmful is when it starts working on your bad habits.

Once you start getting used to bad habits and your subconscious mind also starts believing in them, then your brain starts removing old memories. Once it does that, you might never have a proper recollection of the times you were active. You might remember the day you came first on the track team or scored 3 goals in soccer, since those are profound and impactful memories that the brain loves to preserve. But when it comes to daily routine, you might reflect back and think, "Well, I have always been this way. I don't think I have ever NOT acted in any way other than this way," even though you might have! You were an active person before. If you think hard enough, then you might find instances that showed what an energetic man or woman you were. However, your brain might have erased most of the memories so that you don't have contradicting thoughts about who you are.

Your subconscious mind, along with the phenomenon of hindsight bias, makes you feel like a completely different person.

All because you adopted a few bad habits.

The Difficulty of Creating Good Habits

When your subconscious mind starts believing something, it is quite difficult to change a habit.

Once you form habits, you might end up living with them for quite a while. Your subconscious mind gets used to this idea and the lifestyle you have created for yourself. When you eventually decide to change your lifestyle and incorporate good habits, your subconscious will do everything in its power to convince you otherwise.

At the same time, your brain loves convenience. Taking the longer or challenging route can be stressful. Your brain obviously wants to avoid stressful situations. It's part of the fight or flight instincts kicking in, convincing you that you are better off not trying to face danger. But life is never about easy answers and quick actions. Most of the things that we want in life are usually challenging to get. When you eventually decide to adopt good habits, your brain realizes that there is going to be a lot of work involved. You might have to sacrifice your entertainment, extra sleep, or other comforts that you have added to your life. This idea seems rather frightening to the brain. After all, why give up the good stuff or comfort to go for something else? This is why many people often make a New Year's resolution about hitting the gym, sign up for a membership, and never go back there again. They start their gym sessions in earnest and with much vigor. Eventually, their subconscious minds send them signals, ideas, and memories about all the things they could be doing instead, like binge watching Netflix with a bowl of buttered popcorn. People might ignore these suggestions initially since they have developed an enthusiasm for the gym and the brain feeds off on that enthusiasm. Eventually, when the pain and discomfort begins to settle in, people start thinking about ways to decrease pain and experience more comfort. And that right there, is like giving permission to the subconscious mind to fill your thoughts with ideas of giving up.

Think about it this way. If you really want to make a difference in your life, why wait for a new year? What about the months you have right now? Are you going to throw them away simply because the beginning of the new year has a "starting point" quality to it?

The truth is that people who want to truly create good habits will choose to do it immediately, since they do not want to live with their bad habits anymore. They want to see changes happen as soon as possible, because they know that the more someone gets used to a habit, the more difficult it becomes to move away from it.

Sticking to Good Habits

Plunging yourself into numerous good habits at one time might add a lot of stress to your brain. You might experience a strong sense of withdrawal, where numerous bad habits are trying to lull you back to their domain, which might overwhelm you.

In order to change your lifestyle, here are some ways to inculcate good habits in your life.

You might have known people who, all they want to do is try to attain results as fast as possible.

They start from zero gym sessions to five or six in a week, cut out meat entirely, meditate for 20 minutes every day, go jogging in the morning, and start heading to bed at 9 when they could barely stand 15 minutes in the gym before.

Try and understand your limits. Be aware of your mind's reactions. Each bad habit you are going to get rid of requires a tremendous amount of willpower. So, don't go through them like a bulldozer going through a small building without a proper plan. Start with one habit at a time.

Focus on going to the gym regularly and getting adequate sleep. Since these two are related, they will complement each other. Once you get used to the routine, you can add meditation to your list of new habits. If you find that you have little time to meditate in the morning, you can do it before you head to bed instead. You can adjust your routine so that it fits your schedule comfortably.

For any good habit you want to incorporate into your life, start small and make sure that you get used to one before moving on to the other.

Have you ever noticed how you do not like to get rid of the things you have invested a lot of time and effort into?

Pick up a calendar. Each day you spend perfecting your habits receives an X on the calendar. Over time, you will notice that your calendar is covered with lots of X marks. When you notice this, you will realize that you have put in so much effort into your new habit already. It would be a shame to give it up now. That motivates you to continue with your work even more.

Planning to jog every morning? Keep marking your activity on the calendar until you become hooked.

You might start out by refusing to let go of your bad habits. It might seem that the only reason you are holding on to them is sheer stubbornness. Over time, when you become used to the good habits, that's when an old psychological phenomenon friend comes to pay you a visit; hindsight bias.

You might have started believing in your good habits because you don't want to waste your time and effort, but you will eventually start believing that you wanted to change your bad habits into good because you wanted to. Your brain will start erasing memories of you feeling compelled to change your bad habits. All you might remember is that you started working on your good habits and through sheer determination, you ended up succeeding in incorporating them into your life.

And that is not a bad thing. Why continue to believe that you felt forced to do something? You have good habits now after all. It does not matter how you got here.

Have Clear Goals

When you start creating goals with vague intentions, then you are more than likely not going to follow through because you are not entirely certain how you want to achieve your goals. Here are some examples:

- I am going to go to the gym three times a week.

- I am going to sleep as early as possible and wake up at dawn.

- I will have breakfast in the morning.

Why are the above goals vague? They don't have a plan of action. What does "sleep as early as possible" mean? It could be 8 pm or it could be 6 pm. You could sleep at 8 pm one day and then at 11 pm the next day and still consider it early.

The best way to create new habits is by having a plan of action.

- Form implementation intentions, where you create a series of if/then conditions. For example, "If I wake up early in the morning, then I will do cardio and 10 pushups."

- Once you create the above condition, stack your habits. For example, before I head to the gym in the morning, I am going to get 8 hours of sleep where I head to bed by 9 pm.

- Start scheduling. Once you have a rough outline, create a schedule in your calendar where you note down the time that you are going to head to bed, when you are going to the gym, and the duration you are going to spend there. When you have your plans distilled to accurate timings, you won't continue to rely on wiggle room to allow you to make the endeavor easier.

Some people save rewards for big milestones. The problem with that is that it might take a while for them to reach those milestones.

If you don't reward yourself frequently, then you are going to feel like the journey is not worth it. Every step that you take in your journey is a win, no matter how small it is. For example, making sure that you wake up in the morning to head to the gym is a win. After all, people actively avoid waking up early. You pushing through the fog of sleep and putting your body through a fitness regime is a success in itself.

At the same time, you should not reward yourself too often or it loses its meaning. Your rewarding technique has to be realistic, but motivating.

The best way to do this is to think of the goal you would like to achieve. Then break up that goal into smaller parts. For example, let's say you are aiming for killer abs. You know that you might achieve your ideal body after months of hard work. Ideally, your reward schedule should be done on a weekly basis. This means that if you successfully complete a week's worth of exercise, then you are eligible for a reward. This way, you not only space out the reward at comfortable intervals, but you keep yourself motivated.

Let's look at another example. Imagine that you have decided to wake up at 4 am every day. Currently, you wake up at 8 am and start your day with a hot latte at about 9 am. You are hoping to change that. For your new schedule, you are not going to have your latte unless you have woken up at 4 am for three consecutive days. You are going to stick to black coffee for two days and have your latte on the third day. If you break your routine at any point, then the cycle restarts.

Each cycle is a chance to reinforce your habit. As you continue to reward yourself, you will continue to reinforce the habit. Eventually, it has become a part of your life and your brain will recognize this as well. As for the rest, you can leave it to hindsight bias to make you feel like you were always interested in the habit.

Redesign Your Environment

Remember that we discussed how when people read motivational quotes in the morning, they are priming themselves for the rest of the day? You can do that in this section as well as it is extremely effective in motivating you.

Let's take another example. If you have seen some office spaces (or perhaps your boss's office), then you might notice the presence of plants, paint on the wall, or other forms of decor. The aim of these features is to create an environment that boasts a certain personality. People with plants on their desk or in their offices are aiming for a calm and composed personality, where they are in control of their emotions. Those who have pictures of family or friends on their desk are revealing their values and what matters to them. Each of these objects is a mental reminder.

In a similar manner, surround yourself with items and paraphernalia that supports your habits. If you are planning to start working out regularly at the gym, put up motivational quotes by big muscled men or women who have bodies that look like they could deflect bullets. Keep your exercise gear close to you. You might even have a certain diet regime. If that diet involves meal preparation, then prepare these meals in advance and keep them in the refrigerator to have them ready for your day. All of these little steps contribute towards a mental attitude that will help you achieve your goals.

Create a space that motivates you and supports your work or habits.

Positive Habits Require Positive Thinking

You are about to go on a vacation to Bali. Here are a few situations that I would like to present to you. See if you like any of them.

- You are an adventurer. You love taking risks. It's all about the adrenaline and facing your fears. You enjoy extreme sports. However, I tell you that all you get to do on your vacation is stay in your hotel and relax.

- You are an explorer. You love to see the sights, people, food, and events of the city you visit. To you, the excitement of discovery comes before everything else. I tell you that you are only allowed to visit a restaurant frequented by tourists and nothing else. And maybe a shopping mall.

- You enjoy relaxation. The main purpose of your vacation is to sit back, remove your footwear, and sip on that cocktail while enjoying a lovely book. But guess what? I wake you up at 5 am and tell you that we are going rock climbing!

Would you really enjoy your vacation in any of the three scenarios? Would you have positive emotions when thinking about your trip? In fact, you might not even listen to what I have to say and do what you came to do.

If you do not like something, chances are that you are going to find a way to avoid it. It might happen immediately or it might happen eventually. The same goes with your habits as well. All of the above steps mentioned under "Sticking to Good Habits" try to encourage you to do so. But they will need the assistance of your positive mindset.

Now the important question is; just how do you develop this mindset?

The Power of Positive Thinking

You might think that any subject related to "positive thinking" might be covered mostly by psychologists or life coaches. You might have never thought that the medical community might actually start looking into the topic. But they did, and the results are pretty surprising. According to Mayo Clinic (Mayo Clinic Staff, n.d.), positive thinking provides you with many benefits including:

- Lower rates of depression
- Longer life
- Lower stress levels
- Improved cardiovascular health
- Improved coping skills during times of stress

Of course, a lot of people might say, "How is cardiovascular health involved in all of this?"

Your cardiovascular health depends on a lot of factors. It depends on your diet, the hours of sleep you get, the degree of stress you face, and more. Negative thoughts fuel negative emotions, which in turn causes stress to arise easily in your brain. For example, you are in bad traffic and your thinking is already in a negative state. You are already adding stress to your brain because your thoughts keep conjuring ideas and memories that trigger stress.

Because of that, you might not be able to deal with the traffic well. This means more stress. Which in turn means that you exacerbate your negative emotions. And eventually, you have a cycle.

When your body is under a lot of stress, it increases cholesterol and blood pressure levels. That in turn affects your heart.

Positive thinking is not just essential for good mental health, but contributes to good physical health as well.

How exactly can we create a positive mindset? Let us examine some of the ways.

Tip #1: Start Your Day with Affirmations

The tone you adopt in the morning can dictate how the rest of the day might proceed. Why not set a positive tone for yourself? In fact, have you ever had an experience where you woke up in a state of panic, wondering if you forgot to complete an important task or if you are late for something, only to realize that nothing has happened and it was just your nerves? Or have you woken up once in such a state of stress that you could not even finish the coffee you made for yourself? All of these situations have occurred because when you start your day poorly, the emotions trickle over to the next day. Eventually, you are living in a constant state of stress and negativity. Affirmations are simple phrases that help you focus on positive emotions. Every time you wake up, start the day with phrases like:

- Today, I shall face my day with courage and positivity.

- Today might be challenging, but so is any day of the week. I shall not let these challenges change my perspective of the world and create negativity.

- I am an incredible person and despite today's events, I will not look down on myself.

- Today is going to be a good day.

- I'm going to be awesome and nothing is going to convince me otherwise!

You can always create your own positive affirmations depending on the situation.

Tip #2: Think About the Good Things, No Matter How Small They Are

Don't wait for a big moment to occur in your life. Look at every small event as another positive contribution. Here is the reality of life: no matter how much you want to avoid obstacles, you are going to encounter them every day. Each obstacle is something that has the potential to add to a whole pile of negative things. Eventually, you will feel that your life has too much negativity in it. What you are experiencing is small things that have accumulated to become something intimidating.

The same rule applies with the positive things in your life as well. Keep collecting them, no matter how little they seem. Eventually, the number of positive things will add up to become a dominating presence in your life.

Tip #3: Crank Up Your Humor

Don't let the dark situations get you down. Teach yourself to see the humor in things. Remind yourself that the situation you are in is going to get better eventually. After all, life goes on. Regardless of what happens to whom, life is a continuous ticking clock. So, make a joke out of the things that have happened to you and move on.

Tip #4: Failures Are Lessons

Success finds those people who are not brooding over their failures, but are finding ways to move past them. But the only way that can happen is if they choose to learn from their failures.

You too should approach your failures with tact and wisdom. Let your failures teach you a lesson; do not let them define your life. Bill Gates is defined by the success of Microsoft because he let that be the focus of his attention. If he had let his failures define him, then he would be in a different position rather than on the Forbes list of billionaires.

Tip #5: Watch Out for Negative Self-Talk

It's not unusual for people to berate themselves when they commit an error. How many times have you thought "I shouldn't have done it. I was going to fail anyway" when you tried something and didn't succeed at it? Or you might have thought one of these critical thoughts:

- Why do I even bother with such things anyway?

- What am I doing? I should have just stuck to what I know.

- If only I hadn't tried something new, this wouldn't have happened.

Every time you create a negative statement about yourself, you are forcing your brain to think in a particular manner. And we don't need to go into the details of how your subconscious is going to latch on to those negative thoughts and run with them.

So, what should you do if you are faced with negative self-evaluations? You turn them into positive ones.

Let's say that you tried to do something and it failed. Rather than thinking:

- I shouldn't have tried. This is what happens when you don't stick to what you do.

  Think of it this way:

- So that's what happens if I do it this way! Interesting! I'll remember this and make sure I don't do it this way in the future. Or even if I do, I will plan better. Let's look at my other options.

Notice the difference? In the second response, you acknowledge that a mistake has been made. But you see it in a positive light. You allow it to teach you rather than defeat you. Make sure that you are not denying the fact that you have made a mistake. Denial has its consequences.

What is so bad about denial, you ask?

A lot.

One of the things that denial prevents you from doing is seeking help. We are not all perfect. Sometimes, we need help in our endeavors. That does not mean that we are weak or unskilled. It just means that we might need an extra pair of hands (or more) to help us with our project.

Denial also prevents us from acknowledging problems. If you feel that there are no problems, even when there are, then you won't learn to grow or deal with them. Eventually, those problems worsen and affect your life immensely at a later time.

There are two things you can do with a problem.

You can choose to face it and learn to handle it. Or you can choose to ignore it, and watch it dismantle things in your life.

Among the two options, the ideal choice is obvious.

Focus on the Present

People often misunderstand this advice. They think that by being focused on the present, they have to be aware of every ticking minute that passes by.

That's not true at all. The idea of being in the present – or practicing mindfulness as people like to say – is that you don't let your mind wander toward things of the past or events of the future. The reason for this is that the things of the past have already occurred and there is nothing you can do to change that. But, what about the things that are yet to happen? Use the steps below:

- Step 1: Can you deal with the situation? If yes, move on to Step 2, else move on to Step 5.

- Step 2: Have you already thought of ways to deal with the situation? If yes, move on to Step 5, else move on to Step 3

- Step 3: Can you come up with recommendations, ideas, or solutions to deal with the situation? If you yes, move on to step 4, else go to Step 5.

- Step 4: Do you have a plan of action? If yes, then move to Step 5, else create a plan of action and move to Step 5.

- Step 5: Continue with your day and bring your mind back to the present.

When you allow the past or present to occupy too much of your time in the present, then you might not perform well or achieve much in the present.

Have a Positive Circle of Friends

Let me meet your friends and I can tell you what your future looks like. You might have heard that phrase repeated often. And for good reason. Since it does bear some truth.

When you surround yourself with friends who are positive influences in your life, you in turn improve your positivity.

Take this study conducted by Harvard psychologists as an example (Fowler & Christakis, 2008). The study was conducted over a period of 20 years and the results showed that happiness is greatly influenced by your social circles. In other words, you might very well be the company you keep.

When you surround yourself with positive people, their positivity seeps into your life. You become a sponge, absorbing their attitudes and eventually adding certain quirks to your own personality.

Have friends who support you and accept you for who you are.

Hence, surround yourself with people who help you increase the positivity in your life.

Additionally, you can also find people who can act as your mentors. It could be your parents, siblings, friends, or even grandparents. Being in the company of positive people will allow you to learn from their attitudes. They might even be able to share some of their worldly wisdom with you.

Positive Thoughts Yield Positive Results

Before the 1980s, positive thinking was a concept with no scientific backing. In 1985, two professors of psychology, Michael F. Scheier and Charles S. Carver, published a study that backed the idea that positive thinking leads to positive results.

They created the Life Orientation Test or LOT, revised in 1989 to LOT-R. It was a way of assessing people's level of optimism. It was first used on a group of university students to understand if there was a link between levels of optimism and health. The results showed that students who were more optimistic had fewer physical symptoms.

Since then, positive thinking has drawn a lot more interest from researchers. This has led to the term dispositional optimism, which is what we are working toward. Dispositional optimism is the belief that our future will have more positive events and experiences than negative ones. This type of optimism encourages a great range of well-being benefits, specifically reduced depression, anxiety, and stress.

Being more optimistic and thinking positively doesn't block the stress or worries. It does, however, help you to find the solutions to problems by looking at outcomes in a more favorable way.

So, how does positive thinking lead to positive results? Those with a more positive outlook on life are more determined to achieve their goals. With lower stress levels, they are better at coping with pressure. Setbacks aren't something that stop positive thinkers from achieving their goals. Instead, they will use them as learning experiences.

Here are some ways you can start introducing a little bit of positivity into each day and get more results.

1. Smile

Even if you don't feel happy, smile. When you smile, your brain has a little positivity party. All of our helpful happy hormones like dopamine, serotonin, and endorphins are released. Scientists have also found that smiling is contagious (Hatfield et al., 1992). So, you are also making someone else's day better.

2. Take photos of positive things

An excellent practice is to take one photo a day of something positive. Try to make sure that it is not first thing in the morning, tell yourself that there will be something else more positive to snap later. Something very simple like searching for the most positive thing keeps your mind actively looking for the good in the world.

3. Be nice to someone

Our brains have a handy reward system that treats us to a hit of dopamine. When we are kind to others, our brain rewards us. There is a massive feelgood factor for doing something unexpectedly kind for someone else. Bring your colleague a coffee, a massage for your partner, bake a cake for your parents. Try to include at least one act of kindness every day.

4. Start your conversations with positivity

How many times have you started a conversation with a negative comment about the weather? Begin conversations with a positive statement like "I just heard the most amazing song" instead of "I'm never going to get this work done." The conversation will remain lighter and others will perceive you are more positive.

5. Uncancel your plans

It has been heartbreaking to have so many plans canceled due to the pandemic. From holidays to weddings, most of us have felt like life has been put on hold. It might still be a while before we can go through with our plans but that doesn't mean we can't enjoy a taster.

If you had plans to visit Spain, put on some Flamenco music, make a Spanish omelet, and have a Spanish-themed night.

Keep learning the language so that you are ready for when the day finally comes.

6. Get specific about your goals

Goals are our motivation. Without them, we plod through life with little drive and little to look forward to. Now that you understand that your brain can continue to learn new things and that anything is possible, it's time to reassess your goals with a more can-do attitude.

Think about the things you have always wanted to do and thought were impossible. Be as specific as possible and include dates for when you want to achieve it. Now create a realistic plan for how you can achieve each goal.

Your goals and plans to achieve them should be written down. The list should contain short-term and long-term goals as well as rewards for each. The rewards are essential because they keep us focused and motivate us when times are hard.

Don't forget to keep reassessing your goals so that you know you are on track.

Don't force positivity. But you should force yourself to make an effort to see the good in your life. And if you really can't find anything, it's essential to start planning something good.

Affirmations vs. Positive Self-Talk

Both affirmations and positive self-talk are methods that encourage the mind to become more optimistic, boost self-esteem and confidence, and be even more productive. These methods are a little delusional for some, but science tells us otherwise.

MRI scans show that when a person repeats a positive affirmation, the brain's reward center is activated. Neurons begin to fire and wire to create pathways in the brain making you happier (Social Cognitive and Affective Neuroscience, 2015).

A study of students showed that learning how to turn their negative self-talk into positive self-talk was a life-impacting skill. Students were able to change their perspectives of themselves and others (Chopra, 2012).

Despite the brain being incredibly clever, it isn't able to distinguish between what is real and what is made up. We know this from experience when we watch a horror movie.

The body reacts by increasing the heart rate and tensing muscles even though we are not experiencing what is going on in the scene.

The difference between positive affirmations and positive self-talk is a subtle one. Positive affirmations are short phrases that we repeat, either verbally or in writing. Positive self-talk is a dialogue we have with our subconscious. In both cases, the brain interprets what we say as being real.

A real-life example of how to use affirmations and self-talk would be to start your day with a positive affirmation.

For example, "I have the power to be positive." Throughout the day, you would have conversations with yourself that remind you to look for optimism and, more importantly, to remain positive when things don't go as planned.

I am going to include some examples of affirmations that can also be used as positive self-talk. It's very important that your affirmations and self-talk have meaning to you.

If you read through the list and nothing jumps out at you, you can adapt it so that it is more appealing to you personally or write your own.

If you are creating your own, remember to use the present tense. Just as the brain doesn't decipher between real and made up, it also doesn't react to future tenses. A message about something you will do doesn't cause the brain to react in the moment.

Examples of positive affirmations

- I am worthy of what I desire.

- Good things are coming.

- I am an indestructible powerhouse.

- I am full of energy and joy.

- I rise above.

- I have the energy for all my goals.

- I trust my instincts.

- I see the positives in my life.

Examples of positive self-talk

- This is a thought; this is not my reality. Right now, everything is OK.

- My fear doesn't control me and it doesn't hold me back.

- I haven't reached my goal yet, but I am proud of how far I have come.

- I can learn from this mistake so it doesn't happen again.

- I am in control of my own thoughts, feelings, and actions. These are my responsibilities.

- Each day I am a better version of myself.

- I have the strength and ability to get through this challenge.

- I am a good, kind, smart person who deserves to be happy.

Be sure to make affirmations a part of your routine. You should aim to repeat the affirmation for 3 to 5 minutes, and if possible, 2 or 3 times a day. There is no limit to your positive self-talk. You might need some inspiration before a certain event or task, or it could just be when you are sitting quietly contemplating the world.

If you struggle with positive self-talk, create a persona for your subconscious. Your persona will be determined to fill your mind with negative self-talk. At this point, the negative self-talk won't have the same effects as before and you can put this persona to rest with your positive self-talk.

It sounds like a lot of "self" and this must be selfish, right? Absolutely not! A selfish person is constantly putting their own needs and pleasures in front of others and having no regard for others. Here are what these 3 self-concepts are about:

- **Self-love:** The ability to recognize and appreciate your emotions. It also means putting your physical and mental needs before those of others.

- **Self-care:** Becoming the best version of yourself; looking after yourself so that you are able to look after others.

- **Self-appreciation:** Appreciating that we all have good in us; taking the time to see who we are in this moment.

From here on in, we will combine the 3 into self-care. The reason why selfcare is so important and not selfish is that we all have some form of responsibility.

We have bills to pay, children or parents to take care of, a job, friends who need us. If we don't take care of ourselves, it is impossible to take care of our responsibilities.

When these responsibilities get left behind, we subject ourselves to more stress, pressure, negativity, anxiety, and depression.

Between December 2015 and March 2016, 871 medical students completed self-reports on both their self-care and quality of life. Researchers looked at both physical and psychological stress.

The more self-care the students practiced, the greater the decrease in perceived stress and they were more resilient (Ayala et al., 2018).

The pandemic has also significantly increased the need for self-care as many of our responsibilities have taken a rapid change. Teaching your children from home is a whole different responsibility. Running extra errands for loved ones so they can self-isolate adds strain to your life.

Ideas for self-care are endless and may be personal. Not everyone is going to find 20 minutes in the bathtub as a chance to recharge their batteries. Others would hate the idea of getting a massage or running 5 miles.

Nevertheless, your health depends on implementing as many of the following tips as possible.

1. Eat a well-balanced diet

You don't need to be on a permanent diet. However, fruits and vegetables will provide the nutrients your body needs, carbohydrates give you the energy, and omega-3s (found in fatty fish, nuts, and seeds) are excellent brain food.

Try not to just treat food as a source of fuel. Because of our busy lifestyles, cooking is often seen as an additional burden rather than a task to enjoy. It will be good for your diet and your brain to learn a new recipe each week and have fun at the same time.

2. Exercise

Exercise helps control your weight, improves heart health, and reduces the chances of numerous illnesses and diseases. It reduces stress, boosts happy hormones, and helps with sleep quality.

Both the Mayo Clinic and NHS recommend 150 minutes of moderate aerobic exercise or 75 minutes of vigorous aerobic exercise a week.

Start off small, even if it's just a 10-minute walk each day. You can build on this and gradually make the activity more intense.

3. Get the right amount of sleep

Some people need 8 hours, others do just as well on 6 hours. Create a strong bedtime routine that starts at least half an hour before you need to sleep. As we have said, it might be obvious to say avoid coffee but if you have issues sleeping, you might want to avoid any caffeine after 3 p.m.

Also, as tempted as you are, leave mobile devices out of the bedroom. Screens produce a blue light which prevents melatonin from being produced. Melatonin is the hormone we need to fall asleep.

4. Drink plenty of water

I know that this isn't anything new but understanding the science behind it will motivate you to drink more.

Depending on age and gender, the body is 50 to 75% water. The brain is 85% water. Drinking 7 ounces of water (about 200 ml) an hour can halve the number of mistakes we make.

When hydration falls to less than 2% of body weight, your mood can be affected (Water Plus, n.d.).

5. Take regular breaks

You might think that cramming in hours of work is productive. Most people are only capable of concentrating for up to 90 minutes at a time. After this, it is better to walk away from the desk and the screen for a few minutes.

You may also want to consider changing up your work environment. If you have an area to use a standing desk or if you have phone calls to make, walk around for a while. A sedentary 8 hours of work is draining and terrible for your body.

Drink a glass of water when you wake up and before you go to bed. Set an alarm as a reminder to drink water throughout the day. You can add slices of fruit to a water bottle to add flavor if you get bored of just water.

6. Learn how to say no

If we can't say no, all of our time is going to be filled with things that other people require and self-care gets put off or ignored. Sometimes we have to accept the fact that we can't do everything and stay well. Saying no is not unkind, it's a method of self-protection.

Being assertive will help you say no in a way that doesn't offend the other person and doesn't allow them to try and change your mind. Keep your no short and don't feel the need to justify why you can't do what the other person wants. You can offer a solution or alternative if your schedule allows.

7. Make time for the things you love

Before we became far too serious about life, there were a great number of activities that we loved and made us laugh and feel good. Think back to what you used to do as a child, maybe it was football or basketball practice, rollerblading, or hanging out with your pets.

Look for groups or clubs in your area that offer activities you might want to try. You don't have to make a life-long commitment. But it's great to explore new hobbies and find out what makes you happy now.

8. Get organized

Just one thing like losing your keys in the morning can affect your stress levels for the rest of the day. Forgetting passwords costs you time. Missing meetings and plans is irresponsible.

Getting more organized is a small change that adds structure to your routine and helps you remain in control. Use apps, calendars, and lists to keep yourself organized. Keep the important items that you need every day (like keys, chargers, purses, etc.) in the same place.

It sounds like self-care takes a lot of time and time is already short. You need to schedule in self-care time, even if it's just 30 minutes twice a week or 10 minutes every morning. Make it a solid rule that this time is for you and you only.

What will happen is that you will soon start feeling better and more energized. Things like doing the weekly grocery shop aren't as draining and it gets easier to wake up a little earlier to squeeze in more exercise. You will get more done during the working hours, so you aren't having to work later in the evenings. Self-care is crucial for work-life balance!

Automate Your Positive Thoughts

Remember negativity bias? The ability to remember the bad over the good because each time we relive a bad moment, the neurons in the brain are fired up, get wired together, and become stronger?

If we can use science to break the negativity bias and stop thinking about the negative, we can use the same science to automate positive thinking.

Think of this, you have just had a great night out with friends. You danced, laughed, and this is the best you have felt in a long time. You go home and think about the night. In the morning, you remember a song that you danced to and it makes you smile. During the day, you think about your friend's terrible moves...and you laugh again.

Every time you think about your amazing night out, neurons in the brain are firing and making new memories. If you do the same for all the good things in your life, your memories become more positive.

This isn't just going to help your brain to automatically think more positively. It's going to help with your decision-making and problem-solving skills. We access the memories of our past experiences to resolve current issues. If a friend invited you out and your past experience was a bad one, your decision will be based on this negativity and it's more likely that you say no—limiting your new experiences.

If your brain has the ability to automatically think negatively, it has the ability to automatically think positively. You have to teach it how!

Why and How to Live in the Moment

If you have done any research into negative thinking, you will have seen that almost everybody recommends meditation and for a very good reason. Meditation and mindfulness will help with every issue we have discussed from depression to sleep, intrusive thoughts to stress management.

Like affirmations and positive thinking, meditation may sound like the latest solution to fix all of our problems. But if something has been used for thousands of years, it's hard to deny its effectiveness.

Meditation has been used for centuries as a way of living in the present. By taking time each day to enjoy the here and now, we are not distracted by the worries of our past and future.

Being mindful of the present enables us to stay grounded, reduce stress levels, and helps us cope with our negative thoughts and emotions. It gives us a moment to appreciate the little things in life that can make us happy and the amazing things that are in the world if we look hard enough.

There are plenty of studies to choose from to see the positive impact of mindful meditation to be more in the present. According to Mindful (2018), meditation has been proven to sharpen our focus, improve mental health, strengthen our relationships, and even reduce bias.

The present deserves more credit! It's the only moment we have that has no time. It's what separates our past and future. You will never get this present moment back again. So, how do we start to enjoy the present? Mindful meditation.

1. Dedicate the right amount of time. In the beginning, this will only be a few minutes as you are learning. Make sure you won't be interrupted and turn your phone off.

2. Meditation doesn't have to be sitting down with crossed legs. You can sit, lay, even walk, as long as you are comfortable.

3. Pay attention to your body. Are your muscles relaxed? Do you need to move position so that the tension will be released?

4. Turn your senses to the present. Mindful meditation isn't about silencing the mind, it's about letting the mind pay attention to what is happening. Focus on the light and the heat on your skin. What can you hear and smell?

5. Take a slow deep breath in, allow it to fill all of your belly before you exhale. Keep concentrating on your breathing. Count the breaths if it helps.

6. The mind will start to wander. Don't judge yourself for this, it's normal.

Allow the thought to come and go but don't pay it any unnecessary attention. Visualize it as the thought floats away again.

7. Bring your attention back to your breathing. Each time your mind wanders, accept the thought and return to your breathing.

The goal will be to gradually increase the time you meditate for up to 10 to 20 minutes per day. You can start off by doing a few minutes, 2 or 3 times a day or when you need it. Any time I speak in front of a large group, I will take a few minutes just to be mindful. Don't just give up after a day or two. It can take a few weeks to start noticing the benefits of mindful meditation.

It sounds like a simple practice. But quieting the brain so that you can accept thoughts but not let them take control is a lot harder to master than it sounds. There are also so many different types of meditation that you might need a little help looking for the one that suits you best.

Look at some of the best meditation apps to get you started. Headspace, Aura, and Smiling Mind are three excellent examples. There are also thousands of guided meditation videos online, the voice will help you focus.

A Simple Way to Turn Your Toxic Thoughts into Positive Actions

The toxic thoughts are the nastiest kind of thoughts, whether about yourself or someone else. They provide us with no value, which means the only thing they are going to achieve is self-doubt, negative self-talk, rumination, and negative spiraling.

As your confidence and self-esteem grow, you will have fewer toxic thoughts about yourself. In the meantime, we are going to use these toxic thoughts to motivate us to make the changes we need to see. We can do this by incorporating our toxic thoughts into our positive self-talk. Here are some examples:

- I'm ugly: I'm ugly when I frown so I need to remember to smile more.

- I'm never going to lose this weight: I'm going to increase my aerobic activity by X to lose Y by Z.

- I won't get the promotion because I'm not smart enough: If I take this online course, I can have the same qualifications as my colleagues. If I take two online classes, I will be more qualified.

- I hate the way my friend is always making fun of me: My new thicker skin will prevent my friend's words from hurting me while I learn to be more assertive.

Most people think that anger is a bad emotion. Anger is neither good nor bad, it's what we do with it that makes all the difference. Toxic thoughts can stir up many emotions, pity, shame, guilt, frustration, and disappointment are just a few. What if we could turn a toxic thought into anger and use this anger for good.

Don't let your toxic thoughts cause you to dwell. Get angry about them. Your parents don't have the right to micromanage your life. Your boss can't manipulate you into working overtime. You are not a bad person. Get angry about these things and use this anger to create energy that will push you into action.

When we are angry about something, it is because we care. Global issues like climate change, racism, and gender violence can spark very toxic thoughts. But, instead of assuming that this is the world we live in, wouldn't it be better to get angry and do something about it?

If someone is mistreating you, don't play the victim, don't accept it. Get angry, go for a workout to clear your head, boost all of the necessary hormones and go and tell this person that you won't take it anymore.

Remember that you control your anger, the anger doesn't control you. This technique is left for later on in the book because it would be considered a more advanced technique. You need to be fully aware of your emotions and know how to calm down after getting angry.

If you can't control your emotions, you risk acting on the anger. Only use anger as the kick in the bum to get you into positive action.

For this practice, we need 15 minutes. I know this sounds like a lot but there are still 1,425 minutes in the day to get everything else done. These 15 minutes are going to be the crucial 15 minutes that start your day on the right foot and all you need to do is get up 15 minutes earlier.

Begin by taking a couple of deep breaths. Stretch your muscles, paying close attention to your neck, shoulders, and spine. Now choose a vigorous aerobic exercise such as skipping, jumping jacks, or running on the spot. Choose another low aerobic activity like walking on the spot or dancing.

We are going to do 30 seconds of high impact followed by 1 minute of low impact. Repeat this 4 times. Follow this up with some more stretches. Next, get comfortable and finish off with a few minutes of mindful meditation. Finish off your 15 minutes with a positive affirmation or a gratitude statement.

After a shower and fresh clothes, you will be in the perfect place physically and mentally for the day. If you are already an active person, you might find that you can do more, which is great. The idea right now is to make a start, without the need for any equipment or excuses. Once you make a start and it becomes a part of your routine, you can start making small changes to extend the intensity and time.

Conclusion

People often think that creating a positive frame of mind is rather easy. But in today's busy world, it might not be as easy as they originally thought.

However, I think that all good habits are like learning a new skill. You might find it difficult to learn the skill but that is only because you have been used to a certain lifestyle. Think about it this way; you are used to living with certain bad habits for a long time, even decades for some. Trying to change them in a matter of a few days is going to be truly challenging. Which is why you should focus on using the techniques provided in this book over time. You don't have to start changing all your habits in one go. You might add a lot of unneeded stress in your life this way. While the road ahead might be long, I can say that it will be truly rewarding.

The journey to a good life is paved with many challenges. But those challenges show you the kind of person you are. In fact, when you reach your destination, you might look back and say, "Well, that wasn't so bad now, was it?"

Think about a time when you had experienced a challenge and you were nervous. However, if you were asked to recall the same incident right now, you might talk about it as though it was a story. The entire experience might not bother you and you might scoff at the idea that you were so worried back then.

You see, things are always intimidating when they are up close. It is only when they are viewed from a distance that they seem less frightening.

I also advise you to never worry too much about what others might think. You are on a path to create meaningful changes in your life. You don't have to involve anyone who does not have to be part of the change. It is almost like those times you go to the gym and feel suddenly so self-conscious that you just want to pack up and leave. But there is no need for that. Chances are that everyone in the gym is there to achieve a certain goal. And if they are not encouraging or helping you achieve your goals, then why bother worrying about them? After all, aren't we talking about eliminating the negative here?

So, head out and make a world of change. Do not stop for anything. Make yourself the center of your journey.

It is time to bring more positivity into your life.